Date Due

MAR 6 2009			

An Introductory Guide to
Disease Mapping

An Introductory Guide to Disease Mapping

Andrew B. Lawson
University of Aberdeen, UK

Fiona L. R. Williams
University of Dundee, UK

JOHN WILEY & SONS, LTD
Chichester · New York · Weinheim · Brisbane · Singapore · Toronto

Copyright © 2001 by John Wiley & Sons, Ltd.,
Baffins Lane, Chichester,
West Sussex PO19 1UD, UK

National   01243 779777
International (+44) 1243 779777
e-mail (for orders and customer service enquiries): cs-books@wiley.co.uk
Visit our Home Page on: http://www.wiley.co.uk or http://www.wiley.com

Other Wiley Editorial Offices

John Wiley & Sons, Inc., 605 Third Avenue,
New York, NY 10158-0012, USA

WILEY-VCH Verlag GmbH, Pappelallee 3,
D-69469 Weinheim, Germany

Jacaranda Wiley, Ltd., 33 Park Road, Milton,
Queensland 4064, Australia

John Wiley & Sons (Asia) Pte, Ltd., 2 Clementi Loop #02-01,
Jin Xing Distripark, Singapore 129809

John Wiley & Sons (Canada), Ltd., 22 Worcester Road,
Rexdale, Ontario M9W 1L1, Canada

Library of Congress Cataloguing-in-Publication Data

Lawson, Andrew (Andrew B.)
    An introductory guide to disease mapping/Andrew B. Lawson, Fiona L. R. Williams.
        p. ; cm.
    Includes bibliographical references and index.
    ISBN 0-471-86059-X (cased : alk. paper)
    1. Medical geography—Maps.   2. Public health surveillance.   I. Williams, Fiona.   II. Title
    [DNLM: 1. Topography, Medical—methods.   2. Cluster Analysis.   3. Epidemiologic Methods.
    WB 700 L45d 2001]
    RA792.5 L39 2001
    614.4'2—dc21

                                                                        00–043441

British Library Cataloguing in Publication Data

A catalogue record for this book is available from the British Libary

ISBN 0-471-86059-X

Typeset in 11/13pt Times from the author's disks by Keytec Typesetting Ltd, Bridport, Dorset
Printed and bound in Great Britain by Biddles Ltd, Guildford and King's Lynn
This book is printed on acid-free paper responsibly manufactured from sustainable forestry, in which at least two trees are planted for each one used for paper production.

Contents

1

Introduction

AIMS AND OBJECTIVES OF THE BOOK

The purpose of this book is to provide an introduction to disease mapping. We aim to provide the reader with the skills to construct and to interpret maps showing the distribution of disease. Our primary objective is to supply the reader with an array of tools and skills so that maps may be produced and correctly interpreted. Our secondary objective is to describe the role of disease mapping within epidemiology and to highlight its important role in studies of environmental health and environmental epidemiology.

We have structured this book in a way which we hope is accessible to a wide audience. It is aimed at those with a limited experience of mapping. We introduce new concepts within each chapter and provide examples. The intended audiences for this book are epidemiologists and health scientists within research environments or within public health organizations. Some knowledge of numeracy and statistics is assumed.

WHAT IS DISEASE MAPPING?

To answer the question: 'What is disease mapping?' we must first consider some definitions. The *disease* in *disease mapping* refers to the geographical distribution of a disease within a population. A suitable study for example would be the addresses of people who have Alzheimer's disease in a community. Another example, which has more environmental resonance, would be the geographical distribution of the cases of childhood leukaemia within an area around a nuclear power station. Geographical distribution can be expressed as residential addresses but more commonly, because of confidentiality, the addresses of individuals are not available directly.

Instead, the total numbers of individuals who have the disease of interest within a small region are used. Such regions might be census tracts or postal districts. Morbidity and mortality data are often routinely available for such regions.

The *mapping* in disease mapping refers to the visual representation of the geographical distribution. A map is simply a collection of spatially defined objects.[1] Thus a disease map is simply a collection of disease objects (residential locations of individuals or a summary measure or statistic for specified groups of individuals) in their geographical association. Figures 1.1 and 1.2 show two examples of maps of disease. One is in the form of a case event map and it shows individual cases of disease. The other is a summary map which shows the sum of cases by a defined geographical area: a tract count map. These figures show some of the simplest mapping techniques of disease distribution. In the first example, the map consists of symbols denoting the residential addresses of cases. In the second example the map shows the census tract boundaries and within each tract is displayed the total number of individuals dying from respiratory cancer in that tract. Before any further interpretation can be made or further hypotheses gener-

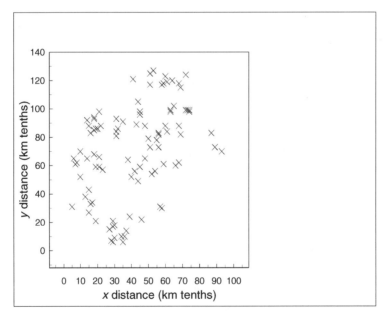

Figure 1.1. Addresses of bronchitis deaths for 1966–76 in an area of eastern Scotland

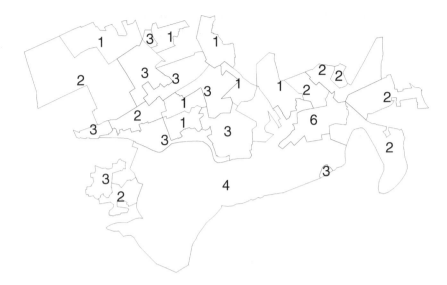

Figure 1.2. Counts of respiratory cancer deaths for 1978–88 in an area of east central Scotland

ated concerning the disease displayed in these maps, it is important to consider how many cases would have been *expected* to be found in the mapped area. In all disease mapping exercises the distribution of the disease (individual cases or groups) has occurred within a population which itself has a spatial distribution. In addition, this population has a variable age and gender structure that also has a spatial expression. To be able to assess whether any particular pattern of disease has arisen by chance, knowledge is required about the pattern that could arise from the underlying population.

The ultimate aim in many studies that use disease mapping is the quantification of the deviation from the background level of disease expected for the community of interest. For example, the main purpose of studies of disease clustering is to establish the presence or otherwise of clusters of disease beyond the background level expected in the population. In a study of the relation between the incidence of disease and the location of sources of putative health hazards (for example incinerators or power stations) it is the incidence in excess of the background incidence in the proximity to a source of pollution which is of interest.

THE ENVIRONMENT, DISEASE AND DISEASE MAPPING: AN HISTORICAL OVERVIEW

'Whoever wishes to investigate medicine properly, should proceed thus: in the first place to consider the seasons of the year, and what effects each of them produces. ... Then the winds, the hot and the cold, especially such as are common to all countries, and then such as are peculiar to each locality. ... In the same manner, when one comes into a city to which he is a stranger, he ought to consider its situation, how it lies as to the winds and the rising of the sun; for its influence is not the same whether it lies to the north or the south, to the rising or to the setting sun... and concerning the waters which the inhabitants use, whether they be marshy and soft, or hard, and running from elevated and rocky situations... and the ground, whether it be naked and deficient in water, or wooded and well watered, and whether it lies in a hollow, confined situation, or is elevated and cold. ....'[2]

With his writings, Hippocrates (born c.460 BC) clearly justifies his position as the first major figure to emphasize the contribution to health of the environment and geographical location. For example, he noted that north-facing cities tended to have inhabitants whose generally robust health was marred by a susceptibility to pleurisy and tonsillitis; whereas cities with southerly exposures, where fog and mist dispersed more readily, appeared to have healthier inhabitants.[3]

Central to the implementation of Hippocratic medicine was the concept of a balance between man and his environment. At this time, the term environment was limited to the personal and general environments;[4] it was not until 1713 that the concept was expanded by Ramazzini to include specifically the occupational environment.

'When a doctor visits a working-class home he should be content to sit on a three-legged stool, if there isn't a gilded chair, and he should take time for his examination; and to the questions recommended by Hippocrates, he should add one more—What is your occupation?'[4]

The potential contribution of geographical methods to the study of disease processes was first emphasised by the pioneer of public health in Europe, Johann Peter Frank (1745–1821) in his book, *System emer vollstandigen medizinischen Polizey*, published in 1779.[5]

'Humane physicians should be set to explore the nature, condition and constitution of the tiniest village. They should investigate its diseases and their causes in the most precise detail, and should calculate the ratios of the sexes to each other, of the various age classes, and of births to deaths. In this way they would prepare for each district a kind of special geography.'[5]

The concept of medical geography was further advanced by the publication in 1792–5 in Leipzig of Leonhard Ludwig Finke's *Versuch emer ailgemeinen medicinisch-praktischen Geographie.* With this book, Finke was the first person to provide a comprehensive description of medical geography. He divided the globe into a number of zones, each consisting of 10 degrees of latitude. He then described the medical geography for all of the countries within each zone. The descriptions consisted of the geographical position of the country, its soil type, and peculiarities of air; ways of life, customs and habits of the inhabitants, and in particular their food preferences; the range of diseases prevalent and the local treatments adopted.[5]

It was in the seventeenth century, however, that one of the first, major, geographically based, statistical studies of disease was undertaken. The author was a London haberdasher, John Graunt. Using data derived from the London Bills of Mortality, Graunt aimed to estimate the proportion of liveborn children who died there before the age of six years. His estimate[6] of 36% mortality proved remarkably accurate, tallying well with later evidence in which the actual age at death was noted on the death record. Graunt's other use for the Bills of Mortality, often called the first modern epidemiological study, was his well-known analysis of the timing of the plague epidemics in London.[2]

Coverage of mortality in England and Wales became significantly more systematic and reliable in 1837, when the General Register Office was established. Its first medical statistician, William Farr, began the task of standardizing the nomenclature and statistical classification of death records. The International Classification of Diseases (ICD) originated from his work. Nowadays, the General Register Office publishes annually mortality statistics based on the criteria defined in the International Classification of Diseases.

The wealth of information contained in these statistical annual reports has been the foundation of many epidemiological investigations. Nevertheless, their full potential for geographical analysis was not fully realized until 1963, when Melvyn Howe produced the first *National Atlas of Disease Mortality in the United Kingdom,*[7] which systematically described the geographical distribution of mortality for several diseases in the counties and towns of Scotland, England and Wales.

DISEASE MAPPING

The concept of disease mapping is not new. In his detailed description of the history of disease mapping, Howe identified several American and British studies dating from the beginning of the 1800s in which maps were employed to demonstrate the distribution of disease.[8] Mostly, these maps portrayed the distributions of infectious diseases such as yellow fever in the United States and contagious fevers in Ireland.

Possibly the most famous uses of mapping in epidemiology were the studies by John Snow of the cholera epidemics in London during the middle of the nineteenth century.[9] At that time, the method of spread and the nature of the cholera *vibrio* were unknown. Through careful observation of his patients and by plotting where the cases lived, Snow was among the first to show clearly that cholera could be spread through a contaminated water supply. His 'dot map' of the residences of the victims of the 1854 cholera epidemic in the Golden Square area of London demonstrated a distinct cluster of cases around the water pump in Broad Street (Figure 1.3).

Later investigations indicated that the pump had become contaminated by faecal material from a case of cholera. When studying the outbreak of cholera in south London during July to October 1854, Snow also perceived that the dual system of water supply to that district constituted a natural experiment in which the question of the contribution of polluted water to the epidemic could be studied epidemiologically:

> 'The pipes of each Company go down all the streets and into nearly all the courts and alleys. In many cases a single house has a supply different from that on either side.... No fewer than three hundred thousand people of both sexes, of every age and occupation, and of every rank and station... were divided into two groups without their knowledge, one group being supplied with water containing the sewage of London and, amongst it, whatever might come from the cholera patients, the other having water quite free from such impurity. No experiment could have been devised which would more thoroughly test the effect of water supply on the progress of cholera.'

Snow obtained the name of the water company supplying each house where a fatal case of cholera had resided. From data held by the water companies, he then calculated the total number of houses supplied by each company in each district. The results showed that the Southwark and Vauxhall Water Company had a death rate from cholera of 315 deaths per 10 000 houses; by contrast, the adjoining districts supplied by the Lambeth Water Company

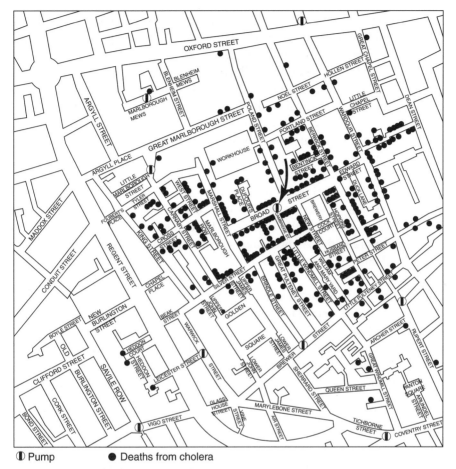

Figure 1.3. Dot map of deaths from cholera in London (the arrow points to the Broad Street pump). Redrawn from Snow (1936)[9] by permission of Oxford University Press

experienced a death rate of only 37 per 10 000 houses, while the rest of London had a rate of 59 per 10 000 houses.[9] The value of Snow's mapping exercises is unquestionable; these studies led to the prevention of cholera epidemics in the United Kingdom.

A comparable use of disease mapping, which included also maps of demographic parameters of aetiological relevance, was shown at the time of the Hamburg cholera epidemic of 1892.[10] Initially, the physicians constructed a 'dot map' showing the cases of cholera in the city of Hamburg and in the adjoining suburb of Altona. They also constructed several others, such as maps of social class, death rates per 1000 inhabitants, morbidity rates per 1000 inhabitants and population per hectare. By showing clearly the demarcation between a high incidence of cholera in Hamburg and a low incidence in Altona, and by indicating that the cholera epidemic was geographically associated with the heavily contaminated water supplied only to Hamburg, the value of the mapping exercise mirrored Snow's original successful work in London.

A less well-known demonstration of the value of disease mapping appeared in the Mortality and Sanitary Record of Newark, New Jersey, published in 1880 by Edgar Holden.[11] It was only after studying that community's distribution of preventable deaths (for example, diarrhoeal diseases, diphtheria, scarlet and yellow fevers, typhoid and smallpox) during the typhoid epidemics of the 1870s that Holden recognized that typhoid was associated more with the absence of sewage systems than with the presence of unavoidable topographical features such as watercourses and elevation above sea level.[12]

The value of mapping in clarifying the aetiology of an infectious disease was demonstrated again in the early 1920s. In a study of the distribution of typhus in Montgomery, Alabama, 'dot maps' were made of the cases reported during 1922–5.[13] By showing that the cases plotted by place of work were more closely clustered than those plotted by residence, the maps indicated that typhus in that locality required close person-to-person contact of people in sizeable groups. Hence, unlike the louse-borne basis of epidemic typhus of the Old World, endemic typhus of the New World depended upon a rodent reservoir, with the rat flea acting as vector for the *Rickettsia mooseri*. Previously, the natural histories of typhus in the Old World and in the New World had been considered identical. However, this exercise in mapping led directly to the formation of the new hypothesis of a rodent-borne disease, which was subsequently confirmed.[13]

The relationship between the environment and some of the infectious diseases was becoming generally accepted by the nineteenth century, and 'dot maps' and mapping in general provided valuable assistance in the identification of causal associations. Nevertheless, the connection between the distribution of the non-infectious diseases and the environment received less recognition. In 1875 and 1882, maps were published showing the distribution of non-infectious disease in England and Wales (and particularly the counties of Cumberland, Westmorland and the Lake District).[14–17] Haviland plotted crude death rates for the 11 registration divisions and the 44 registration counties of England and Wales for several diseases: heart disease, dropsy, female cancer and female phthisis. In addition, he included a detailed geographical description of the coastal and inland boundaries, hydrography, physical geography and geology, population characteristics, and general and local meteorology and climatology. In doing so, he must have been one of the earliest people in more recent times to appreciate fully the potential impact of the environment upon health.

The mapping of disease became more common at the turn of the twentieth century. In Britain, the next landmark in its development was between the World Wars, when Stocks[18–20] produced the first maps of infectious and non-infectious disease in England and Wales which were standardized for differences in age, sex and urbanization. In 1939 Stocks presented maps using the standardized mortality ratio.

Between World War II and the 1960s, the techniques of mapping remained constant, with many of the data being collated, calculated and presented manually. However, the advent of easily operated computers in the late 1960s, with their modern data processing and graphical facilities, allowed the mapping of disease distributions to become almost common-place. Several atlases of disease have been published worldwide; and, excluding those by Howe, four atlases have now been published covering the United Kingdom.[21–24]

DISEASE MAPPING: MODERN DEVELOPMENTS

When epidemiological studies of disease frequency are pursued on a global basis, the dramatic variations in the incidence of many diseases are high-lighted. For example, Segi's list of cancers in 40 countries showed a 12-fold difference in mortality from male oesophageal cancer between the lowest (Guatemala) and highest (Uruguay) countries.[25] (Smith[26] calculated that, if all countries could achieve the rate of the lowest observed incidence for all cancers, the present global incidence of cancer would be reduced by about 80%.) These observations supported the belief that specific environmental factors were strongly implicated in such diseases, and provided justification for the argument that a substantial proportion of cancer is preventable.

Although global analyses can show enormous variations in mortality and incidence, large variations can also be demonstrated within countries. At this geographical scale, mapping is the most effective measure of bringing the epidemiologist's attention to the geographical patterns of those diseases. For example, mapping can highlight those communities experiencing higher rates of mortality or incidence than those of their neighbours. In France, for example, the areas of Brittany and Normandy were found to have rates of oesophageal cancer three times higher than the rates in their neighbouring districts. The remarkable similarity between the maps showing male mortality from this cancer and those from cirrhosis of the liver led to the hypothesis that some form of alcohol might be causing the oesophageal cancer. The French produce a prodigious variety of alcohol: wine in many parts of the country; cider in the west; beer in the north and east; and spirits in the departments of the Nord and Paris. Analysis of the quantities of alcohol consumed by the residents of the various regions of France showed marked variations, with males in Brittany and Normandy having particularly high intakes of alcohol.[27] A unique feature of this area of France is the widespread growing of apples and the production of a spirit called calvados, which is made from these apples. Traditionally, farmers were allowed to produce homemade calvados from private stills. In 1960 however, a law was passed limiting the amount of calvados produced by the farmers; and following the implementation of this law, a dramatic decline was seen in the incidence of cancer of the oesophagus. Variations in disease frequencies within continents or within countries have provided clues about causality in a wide range of diseases including lymphomas in Africa,[28] adult T-cell leukaemia in Japan,[29] and cancers of the oesophagus.[30]

Disease Atlases

Five atlases of mortality and one atlas of cancer incidence have been produced for the United Kingdom in recent times: two describe mortality in the United Kingdom, two describe mortality in England and Wales, and one describes mortality in Scotland. The atlas of cancer incidence covers Scotland only.

The first atlases produced were by Howe in 1963, with an updated version in 1971.[7,8] Two types of map were produced: for 1954–8, 320 communities were mapped; and for 1959–63, 317 large communities were mapped. The work was pioneering, and for the first time showed clearly the differences in mortality experienced throughout the United Kingdom. In particular, the north–south divide in the nation's mortality experience could be clearly seen. Although two groups of years were included, a close analysis of time trends was not possible because the maps of the two periods had differing formats; hence, only broad trends could be interpreted. Nevertheless, the continued poorer mortality records of the north and east were evident.

In the two atlases of mortality for England and Wales,[21,22] the data unit was more detailed than that of Howe:[7] one set of maps (for the common diseases) used the 1366 Local Authority areas as the data unit, while another set (for the rarer diseases) used the 47 counties. These atlases again showed marked variations in the distribution of disease. For example, cancer rates for the breast, ovary, brain, melanoma of the skin, and non-Hodgkin's lymphoma were lower in the north; rates for cancers of the buccal cavity, pharynx, stomach, rectum, cervix and kidney were generally lower in the south. A few pockets of high mortality were evident also: for example, oesophageal cancer in Lancashire, and nasal and bladder cancers in some of the London boroughs. Most importantly, these atlases stimulated the formation of new hypotheses of causation, which were tested both by the authors of the atlases and by other independent researchers.

Gardner and colleagues[31] studied types of industry in areas of high mortality from nasal cancer, and found that nasal cancer was related not only to furniture and leather workers (which was expected), but also that it was related to manufacturing of women's and girls' tailored outerwear. In an independent study prompted by the atlas, Baxter[32] investigated the high mortalities from nasal and bladder cancers in some of the boroughs around London. Through looking at occupation as cited on the death certificate, they were able to confirm occupational links between nasal cancer and woodworking trades, but found no evidence to support an association between nasal cancer and clothing workers. For bladder cancer, Baxter and McDowall[32] did not find an association with the rubber industry, despite having a number of rubber and cable industries within their study area. A census of industries using 2-naphthylamine suggested that these antioxidants were not handled by many of the firms in their study area. However, they confirmed associations between bladder cancer and occupations such as wood workers, engineering fitters and printers. The most novel result of the study was the excess of bladder cancer mortality for road transport drivers, particularly among lorry and van drivers. A tentative hypothesis proposed was that the air of inner cities contains pollutants that may interact with other agents to cause bladder cancer.

Two complementary atlases have been produced for Scotland: the atlas of cancer incidence[24] and the atlas of mortality.[23] The cancer atlas mapped incidence by the 56 government districts. Marked geographical distributions were present for several cancers, but the most notable was the north–south gradient for cancer of the lip in males. The incidence was highest in the north, a finding which the authors attributed to the greater numbers of workers in outdoor occupations and to the reported link between sunlight and lip cancer. Stomach cancer also showed a north–south gradient, although it was less marked than that of lip cancer and the cities of Glasgow and Dundee had high rates. Lung cancer was particularly high in Glasgow and the central belt, but the authors cautioned against assuming this to be a true urban–rural difference, suggesting instead tobacco consumption as the most important factor. Unusually high rates of bladder cancer were found for both sexes in Stirling and Kilmarnock; as neither of these districts has prominent exposure to industries with known occupational carcinogenic hazards, case-control studies could help elucidate causal factors.

The atlas of mortality for Scotland[23] contained several features which distinguished it from previous atlases. Mortality from several diseases was mapped for three quinquennia: 1959–63, 1969–73 and 1979–83; and, owing to the relatively wide categories of ICD rubric mapped, it was possible to make tentative analyses of some time trends. For instance, total mortality showed a consistent geographical pattern throughout the three quinquennia; high mortality in the west and south and low mortality in the north and east. This pattern was similar for coronary heart disease and other heart disease. The patterns for heart disease were unexpected, as together they constitute a major cause of death in Scotland. For the first time the relatively small communities, as well as the larger and more industrial towns were included in an atlas, thereby allowing a more detailed geographical picture to emerge. Finally, several socioeconomic maps were included which permitted the comparison of mortality with socioeconomic parameters.

THE VALUE OF MAPPING: SUMMARY

'Maps provide an efficient and unique method of demonstrating distributions of phenomena in space. Though [maps are] constructed primarily to show facts, to show spatial distributions with an accuracy which cannot be attained in pages of description or statistics, their prime importance is as research tools. They record observations in succinct form; they aid analysis; they stimulate ideas and aid in the formation of working hypotheses; they make it possible to communicate findings.'[8]

Maps answer the question: where? They can reveal spatial patterns not previously recognized or suspected from the examination of a table of statistics. They reveal high risk communities or problem areas, where in-depth studies can be undertaken in the search for causal mechanisms. They can assist health authorities in allocating their limited resources in areas of greatest need.

Interpretation of a map varies, depending on whether it is portraying infectious or non-infectious disease. A map showing the distribution of an infectious disease, especially one with a point source, can be an invaluable guide in suggesting and (in some instances) establishing with precision the point source or cause of the outbreak. On the other hand, while maps showing the spatial distribution of non-infectious diseases are useful in generating hypotheses about disease causation, they are of more limited value in establishing the precise nature of a causal relationship. This is due to the influence of many confounding variables, such as genetics, behavioural characteristics, the difficulty in establishing a dose–response relationship, and the often long latency between the stimulus and the overt response. Nevertheless, such maps are useful in the routine monitoring of the health of communities. In addition to facilitating the generation of hypotheses, and also the analysis of time trends and spatial clustering in communities with stable populations, they can help in the identification of associations between (environmental) factors and disease clusters.

Because maps provide the reader with clear visual impressions of the relationship between disease and geographical location, the impact of the environment on health will be better understood once maps have been constructed for a wide variety of diseases, preferably spanning several decades.

SUMMARY

1. Disease mapping is about the use and interpretation of maps showing the incidence or prevalence of disease.
2. Disease data occur either as individual cases or as groups (or counts) of cases within census tracts.
3. Any disease map must be considered with the appropriate background population which gives rise to the incidence.
4. Maps answer the question: where? They can reveal spatial patterns not easily recognized from lists of statistical data.
5. Maps showing infectious diseases can help elucidate the cause of disease. Maps showing non-infectious diseases may be used to generate hypotheses of disease causation.

REFERENCES

1. Monmonier M (1996). *How to Lie with Maps*, 2nd edn. London: University of Chicago Press.
2. Howe GM (1972). *Man, Environment and Disease in Britain. A Medical Geography through the Ages.* New York: Barnes and Noble.
   (This is an excellent book which descibes clearly and in good detail the relationship between man, disease and the environment.)
3. Davies C (1971). Hippocrates of Cos: the founder of scientific medicine. *History Today.* 273–9.
4. Hunter D (1976). *The Disease of Occupations.* London: Hodder and Stoughton.
5. Rosen G (1953). Leonhard Ludwig Finke and the first medical geography. In: Underwood EA (ed.) *Science, Medicine and History: Essays on the Evolution of Scientific Thought and Medical Practice.* Oxford: Oxford University Press, pp. 186–93.
6. WHO (1967). *International Classification of Disease.* 1965 edn.
7. Howe GM (1963). *National Atlas of Disease Mortality in the United Kingdom.* London: Nelson.
8. Howe GM (1971). The mapping of disease in history. In: Clarke E (ed.) *Modern Methods in the History of Medicine.* London: University of London, Athlone Press, Ch. 20.
9. Snow J (1936). Snow on cholera: being a reprint of two papers. London: The Commonwealth Fund.
10. Deneke T (1895). Nachträgliches zur Hamburger Cholera-Epidemie von 1892. *Münchener Medicinische Wochenschrift* **41**: 957–61.
11. Holden E (1880). Mortality and sanitary record of Newark, NJ [1859–1879]: A report presented to the President and Directors of the Mutual Benefit Life Assurance Company, January 1880. Newark.
12. Galishoff S (1988). *Newark. The Nation's Unhealthiest City 1832–95.* New Brunswick and London: Rutgeers University Press.
13. Lilienfeld AM and Lilienfeld DE (1981). *Foundations of Epidemiology*, 2nd edn. Oxford: Oxford University Press.
14. Haviland A (1892). *The Geographical Distribution of Disease in Great Britain*, 2nd edn. London: Swan Sonnenschein.
15. Haviland A (1888). The geographical distribution of cancerous disease in the British isles. Lancet (18 Feb 1888 onwards): 314–17, 365–7, 412–14, 467–8.
16. Haviland A (1889). The foul Blackwater River in the Farnham district and its deadly work. Lancet 12 October: 756–7.
17. Haviland A (1889). The infrequency of cancer among females in the English Lake District. Lancet 14 September: 534–7.
18. Stocks P (1939). *Distribution in England and Wales of Cancer of Various Organs.* British Empire Cancer Campaign—16th annual report, pp. 308–43.

19. Stocks P (1937). *Distribution in England and Wales of Cancer of Various Organs*. British Empire Cancer Campaign—14th Annual Report, pp. 198–223.
20. Stocks P (1936). *Distribution in England and Wales of Cancer of Various Organs*. 13th Annual Report, pp. 239–280.
21. Gardner MJ, Winter PD, Taylor CP and Acheson ED (1983). *Atlas of Cancer Mortality in England and Wales 1968–1978*. Chichester: John Wiley.
(This was one of the first 'modern' atlases of mortality for England and Wales. The book was strengthened by the inclusion of summary data.)
22. Gardner MJ, Winter PD and Barker DJP (1984). *Atlas of Disease Mortality from Selected Diseases in England and Wales 1968–1978*. Chichester: John Wiley.
23. Lloyd OL, Williams FLR, Berry WG and Florey CD (1987). *An Atlas of Mortality in Scotland*. London: Croom Helm.
(This was the first 'modern' atlas in Scotland; unusally it included maps of socioeconomic variables as well as mortality data.)
24. Kemp I, Boyle P, Smans M and Miur C (eds) (1985). *Atlas of Cancer in Scotland 1975–80: Incidence and Epidemiological Perspective*. Lyon: IARC Scientific Publications.
25. Kurihara M and Aoki KST (1984). *Cancer Mortality Statistics in the World: Commemorative Publication for Professor Mituso Segi*. Nagoya: University of Nagoya Press.
26. Smith A (1988). Computer mapping of cancer incidence. In: Grime LP and Horsley SD (eds). *Medical Geography its Contribution to Community Medicine*. North Western Regional Health Authority, pp. 3–8.
27. Picheral H (1982). Alcohol and a nation's health. *Geographical Magazine* April: 220–4.
28. Burkitt D (1962). A tumour safari in East and Central Africa. *British Journal Cancer* **16**: 379–86.
29. Tominaga S, Kato I and Tajima K (1987). Adult T-cell leukaemia. In: Kurihara M, Aoki K, Miller RW and Muir CS (eds). *Changing Cancer Patterns and Topics in Cancer Epidemiology. Gann Monograph on Cancer Research. No 33*. Tokyo: Japan Scientific Societies Press, pp. 149–56.
30. Day NE (1984). The geographic pathology of cancer of the oespohagus. In: Doll R (ed.) *The Geography of Disease. British Medical Bulletin*. Churchill Livingstone.
31. Gardner MJ, Winter PD and Acheson ED (1982). Variations in cancer mortality among local authority areas in England and Wales: relations with environmental factors and search for causes. *British Medical Journal* **284**: 784–7.
32. Baxter PJ (1986). Occupation and cancer in London: an investigation into nasal and bladder cancer using the *Cancer Atlas*. *British Journal of Industrial Medicine* **43**: 44–9.

2

Visual Perception and Map Construction

HOW TO CONSTRUCT A MAP

THE DATA

The first step in constructing a map is to decide on the data which are to be used and the area which is to be mapped. They may be crude or raw data of disease distribution or could be the result of some statistical processing. For example Figure 2.1 shows an example of a map of the total number of people who died of respiratory cancer within census tracts.

Mapping the distribution of diseases can serve other functions. For example, it may be important to ascribe the gender of the case individual to the case location and to map this function. In that case, it is important to

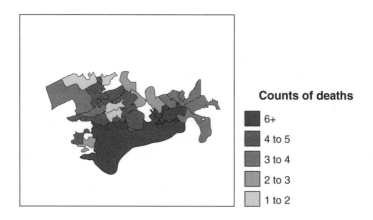

Figure 2.1. Falkirk respiratory cancer thematic map

represent the gender at the location of cases on the map, possibly represented by a 0 or 1, depending on whether a male or female case is considered. In all these examples the basic data for the map must be chosen appropriately.

THE AREA

The area mapped must be chosen with great care. Sometimes this may be predefined. Clearly, a study of the incidence or prevalence of disease in a town, city or country will have as the boundaries, respectively, the town, city or country boundaries. However, sometimes the choice of area to be mapped cannot be made independently of the subject or data of the study. For example, the study of the effect of a putative source of pollution on a population requires the identification of the area to be mapped prior to the mapping process. It is crucial to the success of the study that appropriate study regions are defined. When considering a putative source of pollution, we might consider that an air pollution source (say) might be measurable up to 10 km from the source. If a map is constructed which covers an area much larger than 10 km radius from the source then a dilution effect may be observed. This concept is discussed in more detail in Chapter 5. Similarly, the decision to examine an area which only contains part of the predicted effect range would lead to considerable problems of interpretation. This concept relates closely to the issue of edge effects, which is considered in more depth in Chapter 4.

THE CHOICE OF SCALE

All maps are characterized by the scale chosen to represent the geographical distribution of the disease of interest. The scale of a map determines the extent of aerial coverage possible and the degree to which spatial structures will be observable on the map. The scale determines the visibility of the geographical distribution of the disease in question.

The first consideration in choosing a scale is the relation of the map scale to the study area. If a fixed area is to be used, then the scale employed should represent the variation of the disease within the fixed study region. If, on the other hand, the area to be mapped can depend on the scale chosen then some trade-off between scale and area may be useful. In either instance, the scale chosen must represent the variation within the study area defined. The close relation between scale and area can be seen in Figures 2.1 and 2.2. Figure 2.1 shows the map of lung cancer mortality for Falkirk for the period 1978–83.

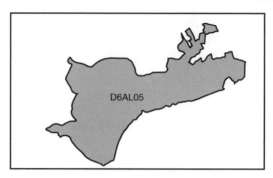

Figure 2.2. Falkirk: single region thematic map

The mortality is displayed as varying counts within enumeration districts which are classified by shade. At this scale, the overall distribution of lung cancer mortality within Falkirk is clear. If we change the scale of the map to increase the resolution (we zoom in to see more detail), we inevitably reduce the geographical area which can be mapped. If, on the other hand, we zoom out to a larger aerial extent (for example, the whole of Scotland) we lose resolution and display less detail about the geographical distribution. Zooming represents a change in scale and concomitant with that change, there are likely to be changes in what we can interpret. Zooming-in allows the examination of smaller areas but this must be coupled with a change in resolution if it is to be of significant benefit. For example, if the 06AL05 tract area of Falkirk was examined, with the same resolution (but with different scale) as the whole map of Falkirk then there would be little information gained from this process (see Figure 2.2). Note also the close relation between the mathematical concepts of differentiation/integration and resolution level.

MAP TRANSFORMATION

After the levels of scale and resolution are chosen, it is common practice to consider what form of symbolic representation should be used to display features on the map. Usually a map is constructed directly from standard spatial coordinate systems, for example longitude–latitude, east–north, etc., and in these instances there is no need to consider different forms of representation. However, in some studies it may be useful to use different representational systems. An example of such a study is the mapping of very large-scale distributions (e.g. world scale), where the projection used will affect the resulting map and hence its interpretation. In that case, a change in coordinate system may be used and so a map transformation results. Although this type of large-scale distortion or coordinate change does not arise frequently in disease mapping, the ability to use different coordinate systems for representation is a useful adjunct to the range of methods available. In some cases, it is possible to use different coordinate systems to better display features of the data to be mapped. Schulman *et al.*[1] have proposed a map projection method which distorts the study region coordinates by the variations in the geographical distribution of the population background. This transformation was proposed in an attempt to 'flatten' the background so that areas of unusual excess of disease risk could be identified. This type of approach can be applied in a variety of situations where two spatially distributed variates which are related to each other are found. However, the interpretation of the resulting map may be made more difficult by the transformation and this aspect of the mapping process should be considered before transformation is pursued.

SYMBOLIC REPRESENTATION

The representation of data via symbols is a standard part of the cartographic process and considerable attention must be given to choosing the appropriate symbols. This is important because it is relatively easy to misrepresent data when inappropriate symbolization is used. Related to this is the use of symbolization to exaggerate or distort the data to highlight features. Monmonier[2] gives a variety of examples where symbols are chosen to emphasize or distort parts of data on maps, where the underlying purpose is to propagandize. This also applies when map transformation is chosen where distortion of coordinate systems can lead to misleading map information.[3]

SYMBOLS

Symbols of relevance to disease mapping can be summarized in the categories of point symbols, line symbols, colour and shading symbols. In addition to the type of symbol chosen, the choice of size and shape of symbol is also important. First, the choice of point or line symbols is usually made to represent discrete objects on maps. On maps of countries urban areas may be points (dots) and lines may represent roads. The size of these symbols may be varied to denote relative sizes of urban areas or grades of road. Point symbols are often used to represent individual events on disease maps. In such instances, a common size of symbol is usually used. Figure 2.1 showed the use of a cross symbol to display residential address location. Clearly, a simple map such as Figure 2.1 does not represent the complete picture of the relative locations of the cases, as it does not relate the addresses to roads or other urban features which could affect the distribution of cases. There could be large areas of industrial land within which no population live and these are not displayed in the map. Hence, although point symbols are used to make simple displays, these displays, by themselves, give a misleading picture of the nature of the distribution.

The size and shape of point symbols may be varied. Different disease distributions may be mapped on the same map by use of different shapes of symbol. For example, the geographical distribution of individual cases of bronchitis and respiratory cancer could be mapped together with the residential address of each case being represented by a (+) for bronchitis and a (×) for respiratory cancer. In addition, the size of symbols can be varied to depict different measurements. For example, if the centre (centroid) of the tract were used alone, instead of the complete tract, to display the cumulative numbers with disease, then different sized symbols may be plotted at the centre location and these can represent the different scale of the number in that tract. Any measure made in the tract can be represented similarly. It is common practice to standardize data by forming a ratio of the count to the expected count in that tract. This ratio, known as a standardized mortality/morbidity ratio (SMR), can also be mapped in this way. Alternatively, if, at each case event location, a measure of some covariate were made (for example a pollution measurement) then that measure could be represented by different sizes of point symbol.

Line symbols are commonly used to depict linear features on maps, and are less often used for disease mapping, except when employed to display contour or surface plots. In these cases, lines of constant thickness are drawn to depict levels of constant effect (contour height), or to depict surface structure along fixed axes (surface plots). The contour plot and perspective view are the most basic method for displaying continuous surfaces. As many of the derived measures made on counts or case events can be specified as continuous surfaces, then these plotting types play an important role in visual display.

CONTOURS

In contour plotting, a continuous surface is measured on a regular grid and these measurements are used to construct a map where variation in the measurement is described by series of contours of equal height. Specifying different contour intervals or grid spacings can usually vary the contouring. Fewer intervals lead to smoother representations. Figures 2.3 and 2.4 display the contour map for two different contour interval specifications for the residential mortality data shown in Figure 1.1 (page 2).

Details of how this density is obtained are discussed in Chapter 6. The contour map can be represented by 5 or 10 (or other numbers) of contours and the resulting map will be altered accordingly. Indeed prior to contouring, the density measurements were computed for a grid mesh based on the

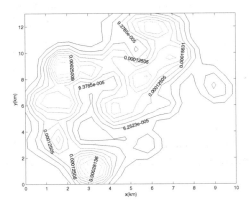

Figure 2.3. Contour plot with 10 intervals of the local density of lung cancer cases: Arbroath

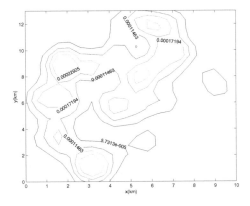

Figure 2.4. Contour plot of 5 intervals of the local density of lung cancer cases: Arbroath

use of a variable smoothing constant. This constant controls the degree of smoothness of the final mesh values. Hence in this case, two stages of smoothing of the density have been used: one stage to give the mesh point values, and the second stage to represent the contour map. This type of further processing of data is discussed more fully in a later section.

Contour maps provide a bird's eye view of a surface. Another possible approach is to use a three-dimensional perspective view of the surface, which highlights visually the peaks and troughs. Figure 2.5 displays a perspective view of the contour surface in Figure 2.3. The advantage of the perspective view is that it allows an immediate impression of the nature of the surface, and hence is useful in exploratory mapping of disease. However, the surface display is limited by the choice of viewing angle and position. By certain tilting, the peaks and troughs can be emphasized or de-emphasized at will. Also much of the structure of the surface can be hidden from sight. Perspective displays can hide more than they show.

COLOUR

The choice of colour or shading schemes is also a consideration when designing a mapped representation. The use of colour or shading to

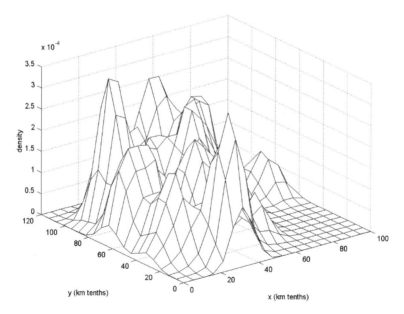

Figure 2.5. Perspective view of the local density of lung cancer cases: Arbroath

represent different levels of effect in map areas is known as choropleth mapping. The use of colour or shading is seldom used in dot or spot mapping or currently in contour or perspective view plots of disease distribution, although these facilities are available in many standard graphical and Geographical Information Systems (GIS) packages. On the other hand, colouring and shading schemes are often found when the data are mapped in summary form. For example, many disease atlases use colour gradation schemes to represent different levels of disease rate within regions.

The idea behind the use of colour schemes or shading to depict disease distribution, is that gradations of colour or shading are easy to comprehend and hence the map information can be received in a simple form. There are however major problems about the interpretation of colour and shading schemes that limit their usefulness. First, the arbitrary application of different colour intensities and colour types can be used to produce a distorted appearance of disease incidence or prevalence. Using bright red for the highest counts of disease on a map immediately produces a visual domination and implicitly suggests concern.

Second, arbitrary scale differences between colour hues or monotone shading are very difficult for individuals to interpret as differences in disease incidence (Figure 2.6). Finally, the considerable differences in tract

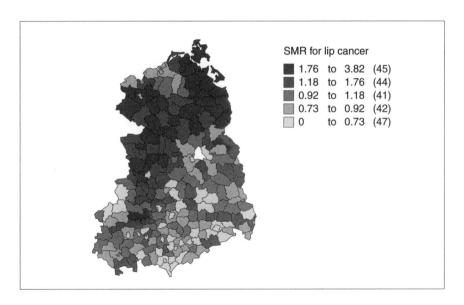

Figure 2.6. Lip cancer SMR map for eastern Germany (1980–1989)

geometry which are commonly found in disease maps, combined with the application of colour gradation, can give misleading impressions as extra and potentially confusing spatial information must be processed by the observer. The addition of colour and shading schemes should be avoided if the resulting map could lead to confusing spatial information for the observer. Many national atlases have been constructed using such colour schemes and such concerns arise in their interpretation.

The application of colour shading to contour plots and perspective views is now possible within graphical and GIS packages.[4] The colouring of contours may help to assess peaks and troughs in a map. However, there is less need for this aid in perspective views, and such colouring/rendering appears to have little but cosmetic attraction.

FURTHER PROCESSING OF DATA

It is sometimes important to consider if there is a need for any further processing of the data prior to map production, and if so, what effect this further processing could have on the resulting map. In many situations, it is simple to conceive of the symbolic representation of the data in map form, and to directly construct the map. Dot maps using simple point symbols or maps of counts displaying count numbers in regions lead to simple maps which do not require further data processing. However, the use of algorithms or procedures which use information between the data measurement points, will lead to further processing of data. For example, the relation between numbers of cases of disease in regions and pollution measured in a network of sites may be examined. In that situation it may be necessary to interpolate the pollution measurements to locations where the numbers of cases are available (such as centroids of regions). Usually the interpolation of data between observed data points requires the use of an algorithm which makes decisions about the best values to use at locations other than those observed. If a continuous surface is to be mapped based on a discrete set of observation points, then interpolation in some form is inevitable. Any contouring or perspective view procedure will employ an interpolation algorithm to estimate the values of the observed variable, usually, to a grid mesh of x–y coordinates which covers the mapped area. From this grid mesh of interpolated values there will be further interpolation to the locations of contour levels (of equal height). This, possibly two-stage process, adds two smoothing stages to the data observed, as interpolation acts as a smoothing operation on the observed data. Many contouring or perspective view packages do not provide details of the interpolation method used and so this stage may be transparent to the users of algorithms. It is therefore useful either to develop specialized algorithms to produce these plots or to investigate the methods used prior to map construction.

INTERPRETATION OF MAPS

The interpretation of maps of disease can have a variety of pitfalls. First, it is natural that the human eye is attracted to bright colours and colour changes. Hence, areas of a map displaying such features may occupy attention. For example, the use of bright red to depict areas of high disease incidence emphasizes these areas, if other colours are subdued. Both colour change and colour attract attention. It is clearly easy to considerably distort map appearance and (potentially) influence map interpretation by the choice of colours used.

The choice of symbol used to depict disease can also distort interpretation either by size or shape differences or appearance of different symbols. The use of coffin symbols, by John Snow, to depict cholera case addresses had an immediate emotive impact.[4] Second, the arrangement of objects on maps has an interpretative impact. It is well established that clusters of objects are picked out by eye more quickly than other features (see References 5 and 6 for example). Hence, attraction to clusters will be fundamental in the interpretation of maps.

Finally, a factor which complicates the interpretation of maps of counts of disease in regions, is the irregular shapes of the regions where counts are found. Differences in both size and shape of regions can affect the appearance of disease incidence. Hence, coloration, symbolization and such regional size/shape differences can lead to many difficulties in interpretation. Recent studies on disease map perception[6] have found that monochrome colour schemes aid interpretation. However, focus group testing has revealed that end-users do not agree with recommended schemes and may 'prefer' schemes which are suboptimal for the interpretation task.

The basic recommendations to ease interpretation for map construction, relate to the simplification of maps and the use of colours and symbols which portray the mapped data as unambiguously as possible. For instance, if levels of relative risk are to be mapped, then a relatively large number of levels should be used (e.g. 10–20). This makes for a more continuous map appearance and reduces the chance of arbitrary smoothing. If colours are used, then monochrome colour schemes are simplest. Use of different colours on maps can be confusing and should be avoided. Try to portray the relative risk data as directly as possible (e.g. display of the relative risk values within each region may be beneficial).

As disease maps are derived from statistical data, it is always sensible to include either an accompanying table of the data used in the map or a second map showing the variability or reliability of the data or estimates (e.g. relative risks) displayed on the map.

In summary, given the difficulties related to visual interpretation, it is always better to inform such interpretation with the data itself, or a second map with additional information (for example a map of variability). An overview of recommendations for disease mapping has been published within a WHO report.[7]

REFERENCES

1. Schulmann S *et al.* (1988). Density equalised map projections: a method for analysing clusters around a fixed point. *Statistics in Medicine* 7: 215–21.
2. Monmonier M (1996). *How to Lie with Maps*, 2nd edn. London: University of Chicago Press.
   (A less detailed recent reference which gives an introduction to the map construction process.)
3. MacEarcheran AM (1995). *How Maps Work: Representation, Visualisation and Design*. Now York: Guildford Press.
   (This book provides a good detailed overview of the general process of map construction.)
4. Walter S (1993). Visual and statistical assessment of spatial clustering in mapped data. *Statistics in Medicine* 12:1275–91.
   (This article provides a good introduction to the effect of different mapping approaches to the visual/psychological interpretation of disease maps.)
5. Ripley BD (1981). *Spatial Statistics*. New York: Wiley.
6. Pickle L and Herman D (1995). Cognitive aspects of statistical mapping. CAM program volume. Working Paper series 18, NCHS Office of Research and Methodology, 323 pp.
7. WHO Report (1999). Appendix In: Lawson AB *et al. Disease Mapping and Risk Assessment for Public Health*. New York: Wiley.

SUMMARY

1. The type and format of data and the study area to be mapped affect the method of mapping. The mapped area should cover the area to represent the process concerned. Edge effects can arise in mapped data.
2. The scale chosen for the map must be appropriate to the study question. The scale chosen relates to the size of study region and resolution level of the map. Increased resolution leads to greater detail. Decreased resolution leads to less detail (smoothing).
3. Symbolic representation relates to the data of the map and the purpose of the map. It also relates closely to the map scale and resolution. Most disease maps use either case location symbols or counts represented as numbers or colour shading within regions. In addition, contour plots or perspective view wire-frame plots are often used to represent continuous surfaces. Choice of symbol, e.g. contour frequency, width, etc., can dramatically affect the visual appearance of maps, as can particular colour scheme choices. A neutral 'let the data speak' approach to such mapping should be made, which puts the minimum of extra symbolic information into the map.
4. Further processing of data can arise due to choice of symbolic representation. Contour plots or perspective views are prepared by graphical packages using their own data processing algorithms which can affect the final map. Awareness should be made of such extra processing. If significant changes to the mapped appearance result, then independent graphical processing should be pursued.
5. Maps should be constructed to display accurately the variations in disease incidence. Given the possible distorting effects of symbol and of colour choice, it is recommended that simple schemes be used. If possible, a map of the values themselves should be made. Accompanying tables with geo-referenced data are a useful aid to interpretation.

3

Data Types and Sources

Chapter 2 described some of the problems typically encountered when constructing maps. Ultimately, how you decide to present data cartographically depends upon two things: the purpose of the study and the availability of the data. If you were interested in the distribution of disease in a country, then mapping by residential address of those with the disease would be unhelpful, as it would lead to an overload of information. It would be more appropriate to use some summary statistic, such as the standardized mortality ratio or standardized registration ratio. However, if you wish to explore the relation between residential proximity to a petrochemical works and ill health, then mapping using residential addresses, the 'dot map', would be ideal.

When reviewing mortality and morbidity within small geographical regions, the numbers suffering from any particular disease are often few, especially if the disease is rare. In such instances it is often impossible to map by address, as displaying data in a way that allows identification of an individual infringes that individual's right to confidentiality (e.g. under the Data Protection Act in the UK). The key problem to overcome in such instances is to identify a suitable geographical area for which data are available but which does not appreciably dilute the population thought to be at risk. A crucial task is to identify all of the sources of data that may be used.

ROUTINELY PUBLISHED STATISTICS: NUMERATOR DATA

NATIONAL STATISTICS OF MORTALITY

National statistics of mortality are derived from the underlying cause of death as described on the death certificate (see Chapter 4). In England and

Wales the data are available from the Office of the National Statistics (ONS); in Scotland the data are published by the Registrar General; and in Ireland the data are published by the Department of Social Services, Northern Ireland. All of these publications of national statistics of mortality include basic information about population and detailed information about cause of death (Table 3.1).

The Office of National Statistics (London) produced a CD-ROM with twentieth-century mortality data for England and Wales between 1901 and 1995, with an update to 1996.[1] The data consist of an aggregated database of deaths by age, sex, year and underlying cause of death which can be used in statistical packages or databases. The CD-ROM uses the most up-to-date revision of the International Classification of Disease, the tenth revision. Basic population data are provided also.

The Office of National Statistics (for England and Wales) can help medical researchers in four main ways. They will provide copies of death certificates for individuals whose date of death is known, or for those who have died from a particular disease. They will provide information about place of birth or other non-confidential information for particular births, or will give notice of all births occurring within a particular place or time frame. The Office of National Statistics can flag individuals and follow them up through time. Lastly, they can identify the current location of known individuals.[2] This service is not free; enquiries should be made to their department of customer services.[2]

A Public Health Common Data Set for England and Wales has been available sine 1990. the most recent publication incorporates the Health of the Nation and Population Health Outcome indicators, and is available on

Table 3.1. Information provided by publications of national statistics of mortality in the UK

Contents	Notes
Population and vital statistics	Summary information for the country
Deaths	Summary information for the country
Deaths by cause	Some summary information but also detailed information by ICD A list
Stillbirths	Summary information for the country
Stillbirths by cause	Detailed information by cause
Infant deaths	Summary information for the country
Infant deaths by cause	Detailed information by cause
Perinatal deaths	Summary and detailed information for the country
Life Tables	By sex and selected age for the country and regions
Meteorological notes	By month and region

CD-ROM for Health Authorities in England. The data include information derived from Hospital Episode Data (HES) and use the tenth revision of the International classification of Disease.[3] In Scotland, this information is produced by the Information and Statistics Division of the Common Services Agency and is available from 1990.[4]

NATIONAL STATISTICS OF MORBIDITY

Morbidity statistics are not collected as a matter of course for many diseases. In the UK routinely collected morbidity data are limited to the cancers and the notifiable diseases (Table 3.2). The cancer registries collect information about all new cases of cancer. Cancer is not a notifiable disease but most hospitals have well organized procedures for notifying the cancer registries of new cases. The data completeness of the more frequent cancers is good; more unusual cancers or those that are difficult to identify is less so.

Cancer morbidity is published annually for England and Wales[5] and for Scotland, the Scottish Cancer Intelligence Unit[6] operates an ad hoc data request service.

The Information and Statistics Division of the Common Services Agency, Scotland, produce a Scottish Morbidity Record Schemes (SMR series) which provide continuously collected information about a range of health outcomes (Table 3.3). The system was upgraded in 1993 when the COP-PISH (Core Patient Profile Information in Scottish Hospitals) SMR project was initiated. A COPPISH record is identifiable to an individual patient, is based on a discrete episode and includes clinical diagnostic and procedural data currently coded in ICD9. The individual SMR records will be subsumed to form a common core data set and items omitted will form speciality specific data sections for instance in maternity, mental health and geriatric long stay.

Table 3.2. Notifiable diseases in the UK

Acute encephalitis/meningitis	Mumps
Acute poliomyelitis	Ophthalmia neonatorum
Cholera	Puerperal fever and pyrexia
Diphtheria	Rubella
Dysentery	Scarlet fever
Erysipelas	Tuberculosis: other
Food poisoning	Tuberculosis: respiratory
Gastroenteritis (babies under 2 year)	Tuberculosis: total
Infective hepatitis	Typhoid and paratyphoid fevers
Measles	Whooping cough

Table 3.3. SMR series (Scotland only)

COPPISH and SMR title series		Comment
SMR0	Scottish outpatient record	New attendances at consultant clinics
SMR1	Inpatient and day case record	Summary information
SMR1 (LS)		SMR1 long stay
SMR2	Maternity discharge record	
SMR11(U)	Neonatal record	Universal
SMR11(E)	Neonatal record	Special care baby unit episode
SMR4	Mental health: inpatient admission/discharge	
SMR6	Scottish cancer registration	Case abstract
SMR20	Scottish cardiac surgery register	
SMR series		
	Scottish stillbirth & neonatal death enquiry from	
AAS	Notification of an abortion	Under section 1 of the Abortion Act 1967
SMR3	Waiting list census	Not named data
SMR30(C)	A&E waiting times survey	
SMR13	Community dental service treatment record	
SMR22	Scottish drug misuse database	Form used by registered medical practitioners
SMR23	Scottish drug misuse database	Form used by registered other agencies and professionals
ISD(RES)L1B	Lower limb amputee referrals	To artificial limb fitting centres

AD HOC PUBLICATIONS

The World Health Organization, International Agency for Research on Cancer and the Office of National Statistics (formerly Office of Population Censuses and Surveys) have worked together to produce ad hoc publications about cancer mortality by occupation and social class.[7] The Registrar General for Scotland produced[8] occupational mortality Tables. Data about occupation were derived from the death certificate and there was concern about the accuracy of the information. Relatives sometimes completed the occupation as the last occupation rather than the occupation in which the deceased had spent the majority of his or her life. Occupation is no longer recorded on the death certificate and therefore these publications will cease.

Various publications are derived from hospital inpatient stays, for example Scottish Health Statistics, Hospital in Patient Enquiry, Hospital Activity Analysis and some aspects of primary care. Some of these report on a sample of the population only and by restricted causes of illness.

ROUTINELY PUBLISHED STATISTICS: DENOMINATOR DATA

NATIONAL POPULATION AND VITAL STATISTICS

The Registrar General Scotland, Office of National Statistics, and the Social Security Office in Northern Ireland publish annual information about population and vital statistics (Table 3.4). For the production of maps, digitized information is available (to purchase) of the boundaries of postcodes and output areas.

CENSUS DATA

A full (100%) census is undertaken every 10 years in the UK: ... 1971, 1981, 1991, 2001. A wide range of demographic data is included in the reports (Table 3.5).

SMALL AREA STATISTICS

Statistics are available for small populations. They are published as small area statistics and are available for enumeration districts (which are groups of postcode units). They are taken from a representative 10% sample of the population. Table 3.6 shows the information which is available for the UK; each country may have additional information available.

Table 3.4. Information provided by publications of national statistics of population and vital statistics in the UK

Contents	Notes
Population	Summary and detailed information
Natural increase and migration	Summary and detailed information
Vital statistics	Birth, stillbirth, marriage and death rates. Detailed and summary information
Marriages	Summary and detailed information
Divorces	Summary and detailed information
Fertility	Fertility, legitimacy and multiple births
Administration	Re-registration of births, adoptions
Parliamentary and local government electors	Overview
Altered boundaries	Overview
Inhabited houses	Overview

Table 3.5. Information available from the full UK census

Age distribution by sex and marital status
Birth, country of
Boarding house, person living in
Boundaries, alterations to
Density, persons per room
Economic activity
Historical Tables of populations
Households, private
        one and two persons over pensionable age
Marital status by age and sex
Persons: in private households
        in non-private establishments
        in hotels and boarding houses
        by country of birth
        by rooms in permanent buildings
Sex distributions of populations
Social class distribution
Socioeconomic distribution

Table 3.6. Information available in the small area statistics

1. All persons present: plus absent residents in private households
2. Lone adults resident in private households of one adult with residents aged 0–15 years, no. of persons aged 0–15 in such households
3. All residents (By age in 5 yr intervals)
4. Private households with residents not in self-contained accommodation; rooms in such household
5. Persons present not in private households
6. Private households with residents; resident 0–15, and aged 60+ females & 65+ males
7. All residents (By nationality)
8. Private households with resident head with different address 1 year before census; residents in such households
9. All residents aged 16 or over (By employment)
10. Private households with dependent children
11. All persons present (By age in 5 yr intervals)
12. Private households with one or more residents of pensionable age
13. All residents aged 16> in employment
14. Residents aged 16> in employment (10% sample)
15. All residents aged 1> with a usual address 1 year before census different from present usual address
16. Residents; private households with residents (100% + 10% sample)
17. All economically active (EA) residents (By age 5 yr intervals)
18. Residents aged 16> in employment (10% sample) (type of work)
19. Private households with residents (Owned/rented, etc.)
20. Residents aged 16 in employment (10% sample) (travel to work)

Table 3.6. (*continued*)

21. Household space, rooms in household space, rooms in hotel and boarding houses	22. Residents aged 18 in employment (10% sample) (qualifications)
23. Private households with residents; residents; cars in households	24. Private households with residents: families of resident persons (10% sample)
25. Private households with residents; rooms in household space (By ownership)	26. Residents, economically active or retired (10% sample)
27. Private households with residents; residents; rooms in household spaces	28. Residents aged 16> in employment (10% sample)
29. Private households with residents	30. Residents in private households, private households (10% sample)
31. Private households with persons present but no residents; persons present; rooms and cars in such households	32. Residents economically active but not in employment (10% sample)
33. Line 1: 1981 private households (1971 pop base); present residents and visitors; rooms. Line 2 1981 private households (1981 op base) present and absent residents; rooms	34. Gaelic speakers by age
35. Private households with residents; residents (By gender)	36. Household type and age of resident
37. Married women in private households of married male plus one married female with or without others	38. Households in permanent buildings
39. Persons <15 in such households	40. Type of household with ages
41. Residents 16> in private households	42. Residents in private households (By age)
43. Private households with residents; residents >16	44. Married women resident in private households (By age)
45. Residents aged 16–24 in private households	46. Residents aged 0–15 in private households
47. Residents in private households	

SPECIALIST DATABASES

AD HOC DATA

Various agencies reproduce data in ad hoc publications. For instance the International Agency for Research on Cancer (IARC) in Lyons produces a CD-ROM which provides information on the incidence and mortality from 25 major cancers for many countries and areas of the world. The data are accessed via a dedicated software program called GLOBOSCAN. The incidence and mortality data are presented in Tables in five age-groups (all ages, 0–14, 15–44, 45–54, 55–64 and 65+). The program is versatile and allows the data to be presented as Tables, graphs, charts or maps. You may also estimate the future cancer burden of your country or region of interest simply by keying in specified trends and population figures. (For more information on this data set email: press@iarc.fr).

The numbers of data sets available on the Web grow almost daily. Table 3.7 lists some of the more comprehensive sites that were found on a quick trawl of the WEB. It provides no more than a glimpse of the data available.

R-CADE

R-cade is a newly available database, which is accessible on the Web since April 1999. It provides access to key statistical data about Europe. Statistics are derived from the European Union Statistical Office (Eurostat), United Nations Educational Scientific and Cultural Organization (Unesco), the International Labour Organization (ILO) and United Nations Industrial Development Organization (UNIDO). Services available include online access to an integrated database via the Internet and World Wide Web, or

Table 3.7. A small selection of databases available on the WEB

Web site	Comment
• http://www.who.int/whosis	• Provides information about all the data collated by the World Health Organization
• http://www.open.gov.uk/gros	• Provides details about the work of the General Registrar for Scotland
• http://www.bizednet.bris.ac.uk/dataserv/onsdata.htm	• Provides information about data collected by the Office of National Statistics (for England and Wales)
• http://hds.essex.ac.uk/gbh.stm	• A large database of British nineteenth- and twentieth-century statistics
• http://www.iarc.fr	• Provides information about databases held by the International Agency for Research on Cancer
• http://europa.eu.int/en/comm/eurostat/serven/part2/2som1.htm	• Provides information about publications, CD-ROMs and databases containing statistical information for member states within the European Union
• http://www-rcade.dur.ac.uk	• Provides information and data about a wide range of European statistics (see Table 3.8)
• http://www.cdc.gov/nchswww/datawh/statab/pubd.htm	• Provides statistical information about health and related topics for the USA
• http://www.uq.net.au/qcopmm/qcopmm.htm	• Provides information about perinatal and obstetric morbidity and mortality in Queensland, New Zealand
• http://www.aihw.gov.au/services/health/nhik.html	• Provides statistical information about health and related topics for Australia
• http://europa.eu.int/en/comm/eurostat/serven/pdf/datab_en.pdf	• For information about databases available in Europe

customized data extraction specific to individual requirements. In the first instance, data will be available, free of charge, to a limited number of academic researchers. An account arrangement has been set up following agreement with Eurostat about highly beneficial bulk licence arrangements for UK researchers. This is a special initiative by Eurostat to widen access to their statistics and to develop a broader base of research and teaching. The new agreement now allows implementation of central funding of accounts and provision of a set of accounts for UK researchers that initially will provide up to 210 data extractions per year from the World Wide Web interface which are free of both usage and data costs.

The accounts are open to all researchers. Priority is given to researchers who are funded by the Economic and Social Research Council (ESRC) in the UK. The accounts apply only to individuals or specific research projects in UK higher-education institutions, and are strictly limited to academic research. Any contract or consultancy work must be undertaken through a separate commercial account.

The database grows continually; in April 1999 information was available on over 60 topics, 14 of which were related to health or population characteristics (Table 3.8).

Table 3.8. Summary of the data available on the r-cade database at April 1999

Subject/Description	Source	Geography	Frequency	From	To
Accommodation and housing	Eurostat	NUTS 2	Annual	1991	1994
Demography					
Inter-regional migration	Eurostat	NUTS 2	Annual	1975	1996
Mortality statistics	Eurostat	NUTS 3	Annual	1977	1996
Population statistics	Eurostat	NUTS 3	Annual	1970	1997
Population	UNESCO	Country	Annual	1950	2050
Population in education	Eurostat	NUTS 2	Annual	1993	1994
Schooling population	UNESCO	Country	Annual	1960	1995
Secondary education by grade	UNESCO	Country	Annual	1960	1995
Tertiary education statistics	UNESCO	Country	Annual	1960	1997
Annual employment statistics	Eurostat	Country	Annual	1983	1997
Personnel in health, number of hospital beds	Eurostat	NUTS 2	Annual	1993	1993
Employment indices	Eurostat	Country	Monthly	1986	1998
Industrial indices	Eurostat	Country	Monthly	1986	1998
Personnel in health, number of hospital beds	Eurostat	NUTS 2	Annual	1993	1993
Road safety statistics	Eurostat	NUTS 2	Annual	1988	1996
Unemployment (general level by source)	ILO	Country	Annual	1969	1994
Employment indices	Eurostat	Country	Monthly	1986	1998
Hourly wage indices in industry	Eurostat	Country	Quarterly	1986	1998

DATA QUALITY

The quality of the data that are used to calculate the rates of morbidity or mortality is crucial to the ultimate usefulness of the research. All routinely published data on mortality in the UK uses the underlying cause of death as the death statistic (see Chapter 4). Yet the reliability of the information on the death certificate is frequently questioned. An editorial in *The Lancet* in 1994 started with the words that 'It should be obvious by now that there are considerable discrepancies between clinical diagnoses and necropsy findings.'[9] The discrepancy was not restricted to the UK but was evident also in Australia, Brazil, India, Japan, Sweden and the former East Germany.[9] Compounding this situation is the practice that necropsy rates are falling worldwide.

It is commonly believed that although the death certificate is probably not all that accurate, it is accurate enough for epidemiological research. However, the evidence for this belief is not reassuring. Early work about cerebrovascular disease found only 65% agreement between necropsy and death certification in New Haven, USA.[10] And the findings were replicated in a study in Edinburgh in the late 1970s.[11][12] More recent scrutiny of the quality of death certification does not alter the picture. There is evidence that diseases are misrepresented on the death certificate. For instance deaths from asthma and chronic obstruction pulmonary disease are mistakenly classified as each other.[13] The discrepancy between the death certificate and necropsy information seems to be around 12%[14] to 18%.[15]

It is likely that the death certificate information is adequate when considering broad categories of disease such as heart disease or accidents. However, if the research is interested in rare diseases and specific cancers then the accuracy of the death certificate may well not be good enough to allow confidence in the research findings.

LINKING DATA

In Scotland and Northern Ireland a system exists (called the Community Health Index, CHI) whereby computer records are automatically generated and maintained of people who have been treated in a hospital within a designated area. In Scotland the designated areas are Health Boards (or groups of adjacent Health Boards) and Northern Ireland constitutes one designated area. Each individual is identifiable by a unique 10 digit number known as the Community Health Index number. The first six digits comprise the person's date of birth (dd/mm/yy). The last four digits are allocated by the CHI system when a person is first registered on it. The first three of these are allocated by sex, even numbers for females and odd numbers for males. The last digit is a check digit. Each CHI number is unique in Scotland, but there is some overlap with the CHI numbers in Northern Ireland. Therefore any study which obtains data from Scotland and Northern Ireland should not rely solely on the CHI number as the identifier. Certain information is obtained and held for each CHI number. Date of birth, sex, current surname, first forename and current address are standard items. Additional information might be held also, such as birth surname, previous surname, postcode, area and district of residence and marital status. More personal, clinical information is also held on the CHI and a security system vets access to this part of the CHI record.

The CHI index is an excellent way of linking health events of individuals. Although available in Scotland it is currently used systematically and comprehensively in only one Health Board.

CONFIDENTIALITY

THE DATA PROTECTION ACT

The Data Protection Act in the UK, is designed to protect the right of living identifiable people. The first Data Protection Act was passed in 1984, but it has been updated by The Data Protection Act of 1998. The later Act received Royal Assent in July 1998 and it is expected to be fully implemented by 24 October 2001. The 1984 Act was designed to protect the rights of individuals when information was stored about them on computer. The 1998 Act has extended the protection as it applies to information held not just in computer systems but also in some manual filing systems. Any information about living people held in a computer or in a manual filing system that is structured in such a way as to make it easy to extract information about particular individuals, is potentially covered by the legislation. All investigators storing personal data on computers, no matter how seemingly innocuous, must register under this Act. (For instance even a simple name and address file of all general practitioners in your Health Board should be registered.) Most universities and institutes have a data protection officer from whom an application form can be obtained. The form requests information about the purpose of the research, the subjects, the type of information collected and the source of the data.

Table 3.9. Key points of the Data Protection Act

🖥	Make sure that all users and uses of the data are properly covered by your registration
💾	Inform patients of the uses of the data when it is collected. They should be given an opportunity to refuse permission
✍	Make sure that everyone involved in the use of the data is aware of the terms of the Data Protection Act
✍	Appoint named individuals to be responsible for contacting patients when permission to use data is needed

SUMMARY

1. When considering mapping of disease, a crucial task is to identify appropriate sources of data.
2. Routinely published statistical data in the UK include: national statistics of mortality (Office of the National Statistics for England and Wales; Registrar General for Scotland; and the Department of Social Services for Northern Ireland).
3. Ad hoc databases are available and are produced by many agencies: International Agency for Research on Cancer; Economic and Social Research Council; and the World Health Organization. The selection of data sets on the Web grows almost daily.
4. In the UK all research using individual patient details *must* be registered under the Data Protection Act 1998.

REFERENCES

1. Twentieth Century Mortality data on CD-ROM [program]. (1998). London: Office of National Statistics.
2. ONS (1998). ONS Services. Contact Bev Botting, ONS,B5/11, 1 Drummond Gate, London SW1V 2QQ.
3. Public Health Common Data Set [program] (1997). Department of Health, and the National Institute of Epidemiology, University of Surrey.
4. Cole S and Arrundale J (1992). Public Health Common Data Set for Scotland. *Health Bulletin* **50/4**: 332–3.
5. OPCS (1981). *Cancer Statistics Registrations in England and Wales 1981*. London: HMSO.

6. ISD (1998). *Scottish Cancer Intelligence Unit, Surveillance Group*. Edinburgh: Common Services Agency.

7. Logan WPD (1972). *Cancer Mortality by Occupation and Social Class 1851–1971*. Lyon: IARC Scientific Publications No 36.

8. Anonymous (1974). *Occupational Mortality*. Edinburgh: HMSO.

9. Editorial (1994). Research after death. *Lancet* 344: 1517–18.

10. Florey CdV, Senter MG and Acheson R (1969). A study of the validity of the diagnosis of stroke in mortality data. II Comparison by computer of autopsy and clinical records with death certificates. *American Journal of Epidemiology* **89**: 15–24.

11. Cameron HM and McGoogan E (1981). A prospective study of 1152 hospital autopsies: I inaccuracies in death certification. *Journal of Pathology* **133**: 273–83.

12. Cameron HM and McGoogan E (1981). A prospective study of 1152 hospital autopsies: II analysis of inaccuracies in clinical diagnoses and their significance. *Journal of Pathology* **133**: 285–300.

13. Smyth ET, Wright SC, Evans AE, Sinnamon DG and MacMahon J (1996). Death from airways obstruction: accuracy of certification in Northern Ireland. *Thorax* **51**(3): 293–7.

14. McKelvie PA (1993). Medical certification of causes of death in an Australian metropolitan hospital. Comparison with autopsy findings and a critical review. *Medical Journal of Australia* **158**(12): 816–18, 820–1.

15. Hoel DG, Ron E, Carter R and Mabuchi K (1993). Influence of death certificate errors on cancer mortality trends. *Journal of the National Cancer Institute* **85**(13): 1063–8.

4

Basic Methods

STANDARDIZATION OF RATES

The recording of disease by geographical area allows the examination of patterns of disease variation. However, maps of disease where the disease alone is displayed (as a dot map or summary map) can be misleading, without reference to the underlying population.

To take account of the distribution of population, a comparison is often made between the observed number of cases of disease and some expected number based upon some standard population. This comparison can be made in a variety of ways and the expected number can be calculated also in a variety of ways. A common approach is to form a ratio of the observed to the expected number. This is usually known as a standardized mortality/morbidity ratio (SMR). Alternatively, one can examine the difference between the observed and the expected. These two approaches represent different basic assumptions about how any disease excess relates to the population background. The formation of such ratios or differences should yield information about how the disease distribution varies in relation to the population over the study region, and thus can yield information about any regions which have unusual disease patterns, for instance high or low numbers compared to expected numbers.

In the following sections we examine different approaches to the calculation of standard rates and their comparison to observed numbers. For the purposes of comparison, it is appropriate at this point to define some notation concerning counts and rates found in small areas. First, we define a study region as consisting of m small areas (enumeration districts, postcode sectors or sub-regions). We define n_i as the number of cases of disease in the ith small area within the study region. In addition, we define the expected rate (number) for the ith small area as e_i. The population for the ith small area is given by p_i.

EXPECTED RATES

A commonly used method for the estimation of the population effect (that is the underlying tendency for the local population to yield cases of disease) is to calculate e_i from a standard set of rates applied to the local area.[1] By applying these standard rates we obtain an estimate of the local expected number of cases for the disease, which can be used in any comparison with n_i, the local disease number. Calculation of this expected number can be made in a variety of ways. For example, if the population of the small area (p_i) can be broken down into sub-classes based on age or gender, then it may be possible to calculate an expected total rate for the disease by combining known rates for the disease in the separate age/gender groups with the sub-group populations.

This calculation can be specified for a wide range of types of sub-groups and definitions of types of rates. One commonly used type of rate is the known rate for the disease available from national records of disease incidence, which are available usually for population sub-groups, such as age and gender. This particular form of rate calculation is known as external or direct standardization. Other forms of rate calculation can be made and these are discussed more fully in references at the end of the chapter.

For the situation where addresses of cases of disease are available, then it is still possible to use standardization. However, usually the expected rates for disease are only available at a higher level of aggregation than the cases (i.e. the rates may be available for census tracts but not at the exact case address locations). As most analyses of case locations are based on the case locations, it is required that the expected rates be computed at these locations also. It is possible to use the background rate for the tract which contains the address location of interest. In that case, it may be required to interpolate the rates to the locations of cases (as the tract expected rates are averaged over the tract). This form of standardization is often referred to as indirect standardization.

CONTROL RATES

The use of sub-group rates is one method of accounting for the underlying population propensity to succumb to the disease of interest. Other approaches may be adopted. First, it may be possible to find a grouping of population which has the same 'at risk' structure as the whole population of concern. For example, if a disease of early childhood were to be examined, such as childhood leukaemia, then it might be appropriate to use the spatial distribution of live births within the study region, to represent the whole population at risk.

Secondly, it is possible to extend this approach to consider the spatial distribution of a control disease which is thought to have a similar 'at risk' structure for the target disease as the population under consideration. The idea is that a disease is chosen which should not display the case disease features of interest, but is matched to the 'at risk' structure of the population. An example of this approach could be the study of respiratory cancer in relation to air pollution sources, where the distribution of respiratory cancer is known from case address locations (rather than small area numbers). It may be possible, in such examples, to compare the spatial distribution of a control disease without a known link with the air pollutant concerned. For example, coronary heart disease may be used as a control for respiratory cancer.[2] In the small area situation, the count of this disease could be used to calculate the expected rates for the case disease, although some adjustment may be required to allow for the different total rates of disease. In the situation where exact address locations of both the case and control diseases are available, then it is possible to calculate an intensity estimate. This is a measure of the local density of events, for the control disease at the case address locations, which can be used in later comparisons. The justification for using control diseases is due to their common population risk structure (affecting similar age/gender groups as respiratory cancer). If using this approach it is important to achieve good matching, as inappropriate matching may lead to considerable interpretational difficulties. In the respiratory cancer example cited previously, coronary heart disease is closely related to smoking behaviour which correlates with respiratory cancer.

THE USE OF DEPRIVATION INDICES AND OTHER COVARIATES

While the calculation of expected rates for small areas helps to account for the 'at risk' population which underlies the disease distribution, there may be other factors which contribute to the disease distribution which are unrelated to the disease variation of interest. For example, we may be interested in the relation of disease incidence to a potential pollution hazard, for instance the location of a waste product incinerator. We might also have available, at the relevant spatial locations, some covariables which relate to the disease distribution, such as social or behavioural measures which describe the local population. These covariables may relate closely to the health status of the local community and so their inclusion in any analysis could help to assess more accurately the local population 'at risk' structure. Often, these covariables are lifestyle or occupational indices which help to indicate, albeit indirectly, the expected incidence of disease. For example, the proportion of unemployed persons living within a small area tract, may relate to the degree of cigarette consumption in the tract, which in turn relates to the risk of respiratory disease. It should be stressed that the use of covariables in this way is different from their use in ecological analysis (Chapter 5), where the relation between covariates and disease incidence is of primary focus. Here, covariates are included to better calculate the null disease risk that is the background at risk structure of the area.

Usually, such covariates are included in analysis via a regression model where parameters are computed for the fit of each covariable. It is more difficult to incorporate covariates in a SMR or SMD (standardized mortality difference) calculation.

An extension of the idea of using individual covariates to help assess the background expected incidence, is the use of composite measures made up of a variety of covariates. An example of such composite measures is a deprivation index. These indices are composite measures of a variety of covariables that represent increased levels of social deprivation. As deprivation often correlates highly with adverse health status, these indices are now used widely in disease mapping. A well-known example of a deprivation index is the Carstairs index.[3] And indices have been constructed also for England and Wales, for example the Jarman index. The Carstairs index combines various indicators from the census returns:

1. Persons in private households living at a density of > 1 person per room as a proportion of all persons in private households.
2. Proportion of economically active males who are seeking work.
3. Proportion of all persons in private households with head of household in social class IV or V.
4. Proportion of all persons in private households with no car.

The end product of the Carstairs index is a single number ranging from -8.48 to $+12.82$. A positive score represents more deprivation. Again, as this index can be regarded as a covariable, it is usually fitted within a regression model where a parameter relating to the index is computed.

STANDARDIZED MORTALITY/MORBIDITY RATIOS

A standardized mortality ratio (SMR) is the ratio of the observed to expected deaths in a community, adjusted for the age and sex distribution. The observed numbers of deaths are counted events. The expected number of deaths may be calculated in two basic ways: either it is the product of the death rates of a standard population and the population of the study community, or it is the product of the death rate in the study community and the standard population.

DEATH CERTIFICATES

The foundation of the SMR is the data of the death certificate. In the UK a death certificate is in three parts.[4] Part 1 asks for information about the deceased such as: name, date and time of death, and place of death. Part 2 asks for the cause directly contributing to the death and about any other significant condition (Example 1). Part 3 asks miscellaneous questions such as: Was a post-mortem carried out? Who was the deceased seen by? Was the death related to pregnancy? If necessary can more information be obtained from the hospital about the death? Were details sent to the procurator fiscal (Scotland only), or the coroner (England and Wales)?

The importance of correctly completing a death certificate cannot be underestimated. The underlying cause of death as reported on the death certificate is used by the government agencies and published in their annual statistical returns. Some plausibility checks are made by the processing agencies, and if necessary a certificate will be returned for amendment to the physician who completed it. However, ultimately epidemiologists using such nationally published data rely on the data being accurately recorded. Generally, deaths of younger persons are more accurately recorded than deaths of older persons. Primarily, this is because older people have multiple pathology and often suffer from several illnesses simultaneously. If the cause of death is rare, and especially if it is a rare disease of the elderly, the accuracy of the death certificate becomes crucial to the validity of the study. Just a few misreported deaths can greatly exaggerate the SMR. In an attempt to minimize this type of bias, it may be appropriate to calculate the SMR for a truncated age group such as 15–64 years, or 15–75 years. Alternatively, carefully searching and verifying every death certificate in the study population may be warranted. However, this approach is not without problems. Because it is impossible to do this sort of data verification for the standard population, the result is, again, an exaggerated SMR. With such data it may be wise to abandon the SMR and instead to calculate an age-specific death rate per 1000 population.

Example 1 Cause of death section from a death certificate

CAUSE OF DEATH

The condition thought to be the 'Underlying Cause of Death' should appear in the lowest completed line of Part 1.

I	I
Disease or condition Directly leading to death*	a..
	due to (or as a consequence of)
Antecedent causes	b ....
Morbid conditions, if any, giving rise to the above cause, the **underlying** condition to be stated first	*due to (or as a consequence of)*
II	**II**
Other significant conditions	....
contributing to the death, but not related to the disease or condition causing it	....

* This does not mean the mode of dying such as heart failure, asthenia, etc; it means the disease or injury or complication which caused death

---

STANDARD POPULATION

When calculating a SMR there are many options on the choice of the reference, or standard, population. A standard population may be anyone that you care to choose. The only requirement is that it is representative of the study population. In practice there are four types of standard population. The World standard population,[5] a European standard population,[6] a standard population which is based on the national figures of the community for which the SMR is calculated and a standard population derived from arbitrary groupings of communities.

There are advantages and disadvantages associated with all standard populations. For example, the world population when used with European data overestimates the population in the younger groups. A world standard population is most appropriate when the aim of the study is a global comparison. A European standard is most appropriate when the comparison is restricted to countries of Western Europe or the European Union. For a study which aims to compare mortality within a country, the national data are the most appropriate. Often a study is more locally based and aims to compare rates within a region or state. Some experts recommend using the relevant regional data for the standard population, others recommend summing the data from each of the communities. For example, if you wanted to compare the SMRs for gastric cancer of Carnoustie, Arbroath and Montrose in the District of Angus, East Scotland, some recommend that the standard population could be the sum of the experience of these three communities. This approach has little to recommend it. A gross and unforeseen mortality experience in one of the communities contributes too much weight in the standard population. This reduces the value of the SMR and may lead to false reassurances about health. A more appropriate standard population would be derived from the data for the whole of Scotland.

When investigating the health of communities it is often prudent to review health over a number of years. Such an approach identifies health trends and minimizes mistakenly interpreting one-off high SMRs as the typical level of health in the community. Calculating SMRs for periods in excess of a decade requires familiarity with the International Classification of Diseases.

INTERNATIONAL CLASSIFICATION OF DISEASES (ICD)

The International Classification of Diseases is a universal system for coding disease. Diseases are classified into one of 17 groups, for example, infectious and parasitic diseases, neoplasms, mental disorders and diseases of the circulatory system. Within each group the diseases are further subdivided (Example 2).

The first ICD was developed by Frenchman Jacques Bertillon for the International Statistical Institute in 1893 and was based on the pioneering work of William Farr who was the first medical statistician of the Registrar General in London.[7] The ICD is now in its tenth revision. Until the ninth revision the ICD was published in two volumes: one volume lists disease by alphabetical order and the other by the ICD number.

Example 2 Derivation of the International Classification of Disease
number for cancer of the lower lobe of the lung using
ICD:9
II Neoplasms 140-239

160–165 MALIGNANT NEOPLASM OF RESPIRATORY AND INTRATHOR-
ACIC ORGANS

162   **Malignant neoplasm of trachea, bronchus and lung** ☞

162.0   Trachea
162.2   Main bronchus
162.3   Upper lobe, bronchus or lung
162.4   Middle lobe, bronchus or lung
162.5   Lower lobe, bronchus or lung
162.8   Other
162.9   Bronchus and lung unspecified

Diseases and fashions change over time and because of this there are differences in how diseases are classified between some editions. The differences may be small or they may be large; either way they must be considered when calculating SMRs over time periods which encompass more than one ICD revision. Publishers of national statistics usually incorporate a correction factor to apply to the new ICD. For instance, the Annual Reports of the Registrar General in Scotland give L tables which contain the correction factors.

With the introduction of the tenth revision, the list of diseases was expanded by over 50% and the ICD codes will be alpha-numeric. The most significant change however is in the rules for the selection of the underlying cause of death. The Office of National Statistics estimates that the introduction of the tenth revision will have a major impact on the proportion of deaths assigned to different disease groups.

THE TENTH ICD REVISION

The tenth revision is likely to be fully implemented by the Office of National Statistics in January 2001 and thus the first routine reports using the ICD:10 will appear in 2002. However, in line with most countries, they are dependent upon the availability of coding software which meets the required standards of the National Centre for Health Statistics in the USA.

MAPS OF VARIABILITY

The use of maps of SMRs or SMDs to represent disease distribution can be useful when wishing to depict the geographical variation of risk for a single disease. However, all maps which are based on statistically computed estimates have a degree of variability associated with them, and this

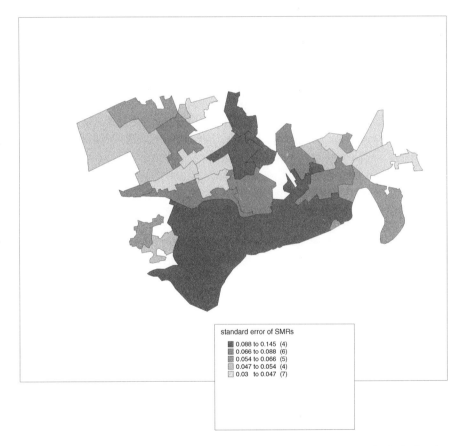

standard error of SMRs

◼ 0.088 to 0.145 (4)
◼ 0.066 to 0.088 (6)
◼ 0.054 to 0.066 (5)
◻ 0.047 to 0.054 (4)
◻ 0.03 to 0.047 (7)

Figure 4.1. Standard errors of SMRs for respiratory cancer in the Falkirk district, central Scotland

variability changes over the mapped area. Hence, we can define a variance or standard error for the local value estimated on the map. Define the mapped value at the ith location as S_i (this could be the SMR or SMD or other relevant measure), and define the variance of this estimate as V_i. The values of V_i will usually also vary with location, and so the reliability of the mapped estimate will vary across the map. It is very important that this variability be represented in its spatial expression, as well as the original mapped estimates. The standard error of an SMR can be computed as $\mathrm{se}(S_i) = \sqrt{V_i} = \sqrt{n_i}/e_i$. Figure 4.1 displays a map of the standard errors of the SMRs for the respiratory cancer map of Falkirk

EDGE EFFECTS

Edges are the external boundaries of the study area, and can have a considerable impact on the estimates displayed on the map. First, when calculations are made for a study area, usually only the data or information found within the study area is used to carry out the calculation. For example, if we were to compute the variability of S_i close the external boundary of the study area, we will usually find that the value is elevated in this region. The reason for this is that there is little information available around the edge regions to make the variability small. This is not important for the calculation of SMRs but can become important when methods are used which 'borrow' information from neighbouring regions or tracts. In Chapter 6, we discuss some such methods.

When surrounding areas are used, the areas outside the boundary are missing and so we have less faith in the estimates immediately bordering this area. In addition, as estimates close to the edge must be based on available data within the study area, then these edge estimates are likely also to be statistically biased (i.e. not accurate). These problems arise when any method is used which borrows information from surrounding areas. For example, in the small area tract case, if averages of SMRs in surrounding areas were used instead of the SMR for an area, then the averages would be prone to such edge effects.

UNOBSERVED EFFECTS

In addition to the use of estimates of expected rates, deprivation indices or covariates, it is still possible for there to be a degree of variability in the observed rates. This can be due to effects that have not been taken account of in the study. For example, there may be particular local effects on disease risk which are unknown and cannot be predicted, a priori, from general considerations of aetiology, or there may be unknown aetiological factors which are undiscovered and may affect the study area. In either case, there could be considerable variation remaining in the disease distribution, which is unexplained by the expected rates and/or covariates included. These effects can be accommodated in analyses by the use of certain advanced methods, as is discussed in Chapter 6. The inclusion of these effects may be important in any study as they can contribute to the accurate estimation of the variability of S_i and hence to the V_i (variability) map.

SUMMARY

1. The rate or incidence of disease in a small area should usually be compared to a reference or expected rate.
2. This reference rate can be calculated from a standard set of rates or from a control surrogate, such as a control disease. Matching of control surrogates is a difficult problem and must be approached with care.
3. The use of covariables in the analysis is recommended. Composite indices, such as the Carstairs index of deprivation, are recommended when allowance must be made for such effects.
4. Simple representation of disease risk in small areas is often constructed from the ratio or difference between observed disease incidence and expected disease incidence. These are called SMRs or SMDs.
5. Any map of SMRs or SMDs should be accompanied by some indication of the variability of the SMR or SMD at the location of interest, otherwise the map may provide misleading information.
6. Edge effects can occur on maps of disease incidence. These occur when information outside the region of interest is required to be used but is unavailable. These effects can be important when estimates in edge areas are to be used.

REFERENCES

1. Inskip H, Beral V, Fraser P and Haskey P (1983). Methods for age-adjustment of rates. *Statistics in Medicine* **2**: 483–93.
2. Lawson ABL and Williams FLR (1994). Armadale: a case study in environmental epidemiology. *Journal of the Royal Statistical Society A* **157**(2): 285–98.
3. Carstairs V and Morris R (1991). *Deprivation and Health in Scotland*. Aberdeen: Aberdeen University Press.
   (This is a very clearly written book which includes the actual deprivation indices.)
4. ONS (1996). *Death Counts. Training Pack*. Office of the National Statistics.
   (The main part of the pack is a 15 minute video that manages to say everything that is important about correctly completing a medical certificate of cause of death. The video is supported by a specimen death certificate, pocket notes, and case studies. An exceptional learning pack.)
5. Kurihara M and Aoki KST (1984). *Cancer Mortality Statistics in the World: Commemorative Publication for Professor Mituso Segi*. Nagoya: University of Nagoya Press.
6. Waterhouse J, Muir C and Correa PJP (1982). *Cancer Incidence in Five Continents*, volume 4. IARC (Lyons).
   (This book provides all of the raw data for undertaking your own analyses.)
7. WHO (1977). *Manual of the International Statistical Classification of Diseases, Injuries and Causes of Death*. Geneva: WHO.

5

Study Design

OVERVIEW

In most studies investigating the geographical distribution of disease, there is a need to consider many issues about the study design, such as: definition of the study area, its size and shape, time period, choice of disease for study, choice of controls and covariates (if appropriate). Generally the purpose of the study guides many of the decisions made about these issues. However, sometimes the decisions are tempered by external factors to the study. For example, if the aim of the work is to map the contemporaneous distribution of health services in a Health Board region, then the study region, subject (Health Service) and time period are predefined. The decisions remaining about study design are minor and may only include issues of population density or communication networks.

If the aim of the study, however, is to monitor the health of communities within a Health Board, the complexities of the study design are appreciable. The geographical unit is clearly dictated by the purpose of the study and perhaps also the time period. But considerable thought must be given to the rest of the study design. Which diseases are to be monitored? And if the aim is to evaluate the health of a community should all major diseases be included or only those with significant public health importance or those with high financial burden? Who should be monitored? Should the health of populations be described by age and by sex? What other characteristics should be monitored which might have local rather than national significance? How should the diseases be represented—as relative risks, standardized mortality/morbidity ratios or as age-specific rates? Should the rates be age-truncated? Which geographical unit is appropriate?

DISEASE MAPPING

The choice of which geographical unit to use in the presentation or statistical analysis of data is fraught with difficulties. Often the choice of geographical unit is defined by the availability of data rather than by the need of the study. Routine statistics are commonly available by towns; but often this level of unit is too broad for epidemiological or Health Board interest. The smallest data unit for which health data are routinely available is the postcode sector (in the UK). The level of aggregation chosen must be considered very carefully.

ECOLOGICAL STUDIES

In ecological studies of the relation between the presence of disease and explanatory variables, there is usually greater freedom (and thus a greater potential for error) in the choice of study area, time period and other design factors. These studies are not primarily intended to provide precise geographical information about disease but are focused on investigating the relation between incidence and explanatory variables. The concerns affecting study design are often about elucidation and identification of appropriate explanatory variables, data quality and appropriate statistical analysis. In an ecological study of the relation between, for example, the incidence of cardiovascular disease and environmental and lifestyle variables, the main concerns might include: data quality, choice of geographical unit, and appropriate statistical analysis and interpretation. How accurate is the recording of cardiovascular events in hospital? Are registers of cardiovascular diseases maintained in all regions of the study area? Are the registers maintained to the same standard across the study area? Is the same information about the explanatory variables collected with the same thoroughness throughout the study area? In the data analysis can different aggregation levels be incorporated, or can unobserved variables be accommodated within the analysis?

The choice of study area for ecological studies is constrained by the need to provide statistically reliable results. For example, a study area with only 10 sub-regions where counts of (especially rare) diseases are available provides little reliability in results compared to a study with 500 sub-regions. The criterion of size also applies to situations where the locations of cases by address are available. In addition, it is probably important to design a study area so that the full range of variation in counts and covariables is included. A study of disease that was confined to areas of high incidence would ignore the perhaps different relation found in lower incidence areas. Similarly, confining a study to areas with a particular value of a covariable prevents the study from describing the full extent of the relation between the disease and that covariable. The choice of geographical aggregation at which the disease incidence is examined affects the nature of the inference possible. Using counts of disease within large administrative regions limits the inference to areas of that level of aggregation. Aggregation to large units inevitably loses spatial information which could help to identify relations more clearly. In general, the smallest level of geographical aggregation suitable for the study should be used.

STUDIES OF DISEASE CLUSTERING

When investigating disease clustering, the identification of the appropriate study area is central to the success of the study. Ultimately, the aim of clustering investigations is to assess whether a disease truly clusters within a region. Specifically, clustering studies aim to identify whether there is disease clustering within the study area; to assess the nature of the overall clustering (that is the scale or degree of its occurrence); and, to identify the location of clusters within the study area. Knowledge is required about the expected form that the disease clustering may take so that an appropriate global cluster analysis method can be used. When trying to assess the number and spatial location of clusters great care must be taken in the choice of study area. The locational assessment of clusters is affected greatly by the edge effect problem (see Chapter 4). Clusters may be only partially observed in the boundary region of the study area if the study area is not correctly identified.

PUTATIVE SOURCES OF HAZARD

Perhaps the greatest effect of study design on the outcome of a study is with the analysis of point sources of a putative health hazard. The aim of these studies is typically to assess health status within the vicinity of the point source. Often this location is regarded as the centre of a cluster of cases, and the relation between disease occurrence and explanatory variables such as exposure measurements or surrogates such as distance and direction around the source, is to be assessed. In such studies approaches using elements of cluster and ecological analysis are often appropriate. It is often very difficult to define precise geographical and temporal windows within which to study a population's health status. The following sections focus attention on key aspects of the design of such studies.

IDENTIFICATION OF THE STUDY AREA

When investigating a problem of potential environmental origin it is vital to delineate accurately the exposed population and non-exposed population. There are several ways in which this can be achieved but the aim is the same for each, and is to permit the identification, a priori, of the areas at primary risk from the putative source of pollution. Many researchers arbitrarily assign concentric areas using the putative source of pollution as the epicentre.[1,2] This approach has difficulties as it inevitably leads to dilution of the health effect. The following example illustrates this point. In the late 1980s there was public concern about possible pollution emanating from a chemical waste incinerator in central Scotland. An independent review group was set up by the Scottish Office[1] and asked to investigate the claims of animal and human ill health in the area. The review group defined their study area by using the incinerator as the epicentre of a circle with a radius of 5 km. This area covered 78.6 km^2 and encompassed a population of 38 000. The town in which the chemical incinerator was situated had a population of about 9000 at the time. The potential was appreciable for dilution of the health effect of living next to the incinerator.

An alternative method of identifying the population at risk is to choose the area with due reference to all factors which may influence the spread of pollutants emanating from the putative source. While the factors vary with each investigation the researcher should consider physical characteristics such as prevailing wind direction and local topography, and population characteristics such as the level of social deprivation.

PREVAILING WIND DIRECTION

The study area must be identified using local knowledge about the meteorological peculiarities that may exist. The importance of this point is illustrated by the example of the Seveso accident. In July 1976, a chemical reactor exploded at the ICMESA (Industrie Chimiche Meda Societa Anonima) chemical plant in Seveso, northern Italy. A toxic cloud formed which was heavily contaminated by TCDD (2,3,7,8-tetrachlorodibenzo-p-dioxin). In identifying their study area, the epidemiologists ascertained the wind direction at the time of the explosion (it was a mild southerly breeze), and undertook detailed soil sampling for the presence of TCDDs. On the basis of their findings, they identified a total study area about 5 km long and 700 m wide,[3,4] which contained three zones representing differing risks of exposure to pollution (Figure 5.1): a zone of immediate risk (zone A), a zone of secondary risk (zone B) and a zone of least contamination (zone R). Had these epidemiologists adopted an arbitrary circular approach, epidemiological dilution would have resulted (as shown by the circle around the study area in Figure 5.1).

In the UK the winds from the southwest are predominant with a frequency of about 25–30%; however, these winds are usually turbulent and therefore tend to disperse and dilute plumes from sources of pollution. The next most common winds (15–20%) are from the northeast; these winds are more frequently gentle and associated with anticyclonic conditions and temperature inversions. Temperature inversions are formed when the air is prevented from rising by a layer of warmer air above; inversions lead to the trapping

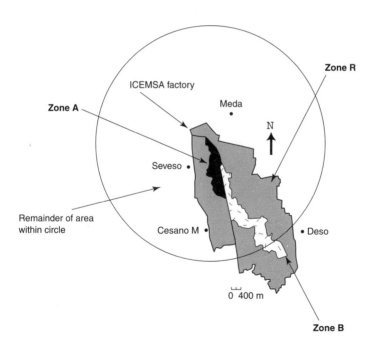

Figure 5.1. Map showing the Seveso area and three zones at differing risks of airborne pollution with a circle of a radius of 5 km superimposed. Adapted from Bertazzi et al. 1989[27]

of airborne pollution close to the ground. The frequencies of haze, mist and fog are useful meteorological parameters for indicating the accumulation of pollutants in the stagnant air. In the UK, haze, mist and fog (whether in winter or in summer) are more associated with winds from the northeast than with winds from any other direction.

UMBRELLA EFFECT

The spread of airborne pollution is determined by both geographical and physical properties. The height and width of the chimney affect the distance the plume can travel. A short, fat chimney results in a slow velocity and keeps the pollution close to the chimney stack. By contrast, a tall narrow chimney pushes the plume high into the sky and the pollution fallout is at some distance from the stack. The 'umbrella effect' describes the apparent protection of the immediate surroundings of the chimney stack. Also, only heavy particles settle out quickly from the plume, while the lighter more pathogenic pollutants take longer.

TOPOGRAPHY

The local topography can have an appreciable effect both on the dispersal of plumes emanating from chimneys and on the interpretation of mortality and morbidity data.

The effect of valleys and mountains on the dispersal of airborne pollution is well documented. Valleys can lead to the channelling of air pollution and mountains can act as brakes on the flow of pollution. The impact of buildings and vegetation is often overlooked. For instance, high buildings, such as tenements and office blocks, can channel airborne pollution in unexpected directions; and a screen of densely packed conifers can act likewise.

Interpretation of mortality and morbidity data must be done with knowledge of local topography. For example the age of the housing stock can have a marked effect on how the data are interpreted. New housing on a tightly packed housing development often has a high proportion of young couples bringing up children. Such a community would have quite a different exposure risk from a more middle-aged commuter community, where the couple worked away from home. Children playing in gardens are particularly vulnerable to exposure. First, their age and size render them more susceptible to the effect of pollutants. Second, they often get a double dose of exposure, through the air and also through contact with the soil.

It is also important to check that the residents in the new housing estate have lived in their homes long enough to have had sufficient exposure.

Knowledge of the use of housing in the community is important. A cluster of deaths in a part of the community may be the consequence of exposure, but it could also be the site of a residential nursing home. (The address cited on the death certificate is the last residence of the deceased— hence a nursing home may masquerade as an exciting cluster of disease to the unwary.)

TIME SCALE

The time scale of an investigation is dictated by its aims. However, whenever possible it is important to try and obtain some information for the community which can act as baseline data. Thus, information should be collected about the health of the community before the pollutant was released. Ideally, monitoring of the health should be done prospectively so that the biases of a retrospective study may be avoided.

If the disease is rare or the community small, a low number of events may lead to exaggerated variability in the data. To avoid this it is usual to add together the events for a number of years. The choice of years is important. For instance, if levels of the pollutant are not measured contemporaneously it is vital that the groups of years selected should reflect similar levels of exposure to the pollutant.

If the disease of interest is a cancer, it is advisable to allow for several follow-up studies. Cancer latency varies between and within the many categories of cancer. For instance, the latency of lung cancer, assuming smoking as the cause of the disease, is quoted invariably as about 20 years. However, some researchers suggest that the latency may reduce to as little as 5 years if the person is both a smoker and exposed to specific environmental promoters.[5] The latency period for any given cancer is likely to be dependent on many factors, only some of which will be known to the researchers. Follow-up studies should be planned at regular intervals (say every 5 or 10 years) until there is certainty that the cancer incidence is not affected.

DISEASES TO BE MONITORED

Different pollutants target different organs and systems,[6] therefore, the type of pollution dictates the disease(s) to be monitored. Toxicity can vary between men and women,[7] between young and old and between the sick and healthy.[8] Examples of the range of systems affected and major health outcomes associated with exposure to some pollutants are shown in Table 5.1. This is a very simple table and shows only those associations which have been demonstrated unequivocally to be causally related.

Unless the nature of the contaminant is clear-cut, as with TCDDs in Seveso[4] and radioactivity in Chernobyl,[9] a degree of educated guesswork is necessary when selecting the diseases to be monitored.

CHANGES IN DISEASE NOTIFICATION

When investigating time trends of disease it is important to remember about the change in disease notification which may occur between ICD revisions. This impacts on how you retrieve data from national statistics. As mentioned in Chapter 4, most publishers of national statistics incorporate a correction factor to apply to the current data set. Another factor which should be considered is changes which are due to diagnostic fashion. For example, national statistics in the UK show that the incidence of asthma is increasing. However, it is not clear whether this is due to a true change in the incidence rate or to a change in the willingness to diagnose the disease.

TYPE OF STUDY

There are several possible study designs which may be used for investigating the health consequences of living near to sources of pollution. The most common, in order of their methodological robustness, are: cohort studies,

Table 5.1. Systems affected and health outcomes of selected pollutants

Pollutant	System	Health outcome
Organophosphate pesticides	Central nervous system	Impaired: visual memory, dexterity, problem solving
Nickel	Respiratory	Lung and nasal cancer
	Reproductive	Fetal deformities
Radiation	Haematopoietic	Leukaemia
Dioxin	Skin	Chloracne
Sulphur dioxide	Respiratory	Exacerbates chronic bronchitis and possibly asthma
Benzene	Haematopoietic	Leukaemia
Lead	Haematopoeitic	Haem synthesis
	Central nervous system	Children's IQ
	Endocrine	Enzyme malfunction
Asbestos	Respiratory	Asbestosis, mesothelioma, lung cancer

case-control studies, before and after studies, and cross-sectional studies. These study designs will be mentioned only briefly as they are well described in standard epidemiological textbooks.

The cohort study design is the most robust. It compares frequency of disease in the exposed and non-exposed populations. Because the data are collected prospectively, the study is not hindered by the bias of recall and detailed health data may be collected. Case-control studies are frequently used in exposure studies. In these types of studies the frequency of exposure is compared between cases and controls. Case-control studies are fairly robust but recall of events may be a problem and may bias the data. Before and after studies are sometimes used in exposure studies and especially when the research is undertaken when the putative hazard has known to have stopped. A major difficulty with this type of study is obtaining sufficiently detailed and relevant data about the health of a community before the polluting source was active. Additionally, any questioning of a community about its health status before exposure to the source of pollution is likely to be biased. Cross-sectional studies are the least robust study design. This approach gives a one-off snapshot of the health status of a community. The data may not be representative and interpretation of the study findings must be done with care.

It is important to collect as much information as possible about the levels of exposure. Questions which your research should try to answer include:

- Can exposure be reliably ascertained and verified?
- Can a non-exposed population be examined? If so, can this group be selected from the same population as the exposed?
- What factors (other than exposure) may affect the postulated health outcome?
- Are the exposed and non-exposed populations similar in respect of confounding factors?
- Can a dose–response relationship be shown between exposure and health outcome?
- Is the follow-up long enough for the health outcomes to occur?
- Are there sufficient numbers of exposed and non-exposed people to investigate?

CRITERIA FOR CAUSATION

A key goal for your study is the establishment of cause and effect between a (putative) pollution source and ill health. A major problem for achieving this is that chemicals are often produced by a variety of sources. For instance, although municipal waste incineration produces at least 25 noxious groups of chemicals: antimony, arsenic, beryllium, cadmium, carbon monoxide, chromium, cobalt, copper, dioxins and furans, hydrogen chloride, hydrogen fluoride, lead, magnesium, mercury, nickel, nitrogen oxides, particulates, polycyclic aromatic hydrocarbons, polychlorinated biphenyls, selenium, sulphur dioxide, thallium, tin, vanadium and zinc, these chemicals are produced also by a variety of other sources. Nineteen of these 25 chemicals are constituents of tobacco smoke, 10 of the 25 are liberated through burning coal, and 6 of the 25 are found in exhaust emissions from motor vehicles. Municipal waste incineration is the major contributor of 9 of the 25 chemicals. All of these chemicals occur at background levels in the environment. Confirmation of an unequivocal association between incineration and an adverse environmental or human health impact is thus extremely difficult.

Several authors[10–12] have suggested criteria to help investigators assess whether or not they have found a true relationship between exposure and a health outcome. The most famous of these criteria are those described by Bradford Hill.[11] He proposed eight criteria:

1. **Strength.** How strong is the association between the exposure and the health outcome? The classic example of these criteria is Percival Potts' study of chimney sweeps and scrotal cancer. At the turn of the twentieth century, chimney sweeps were exposed to tar and mineral oils. Their incidence of scrotal cancer was about 200 times higher than that of people not exposed to such chemicals. Strength of association is often measured by the relative risk.

2. **Consistency.** How consistent is the observed outcome? For example, is the outcome observed in other people, in different places, circumstances and time? Do retrospective and prospective studies show the same outcome? Consistency is an important concept but it is not always easily interpreted. For instance, the association between smoking and lung cancer is consistently found in studies of all types: case-control,[13,14] cohort,[15,16] and also between various age-groups[17] and the sexes. The main reason why the lung cancer and smoking model is so consistent is because the incidence of lung cancer in the general population is almost entirely due to exposure to tobacco. Consistency in environmental studies is often much more difficult to demonstrate because of the multifactorial nature of the outcome and exposure. The example of the multiplicity of by-products of municipal waste incineration is a good

example. Because of the diversity of by-products, consistency of results between different incinerators may be difficult to achieve.

3. **Specificity.** This criterion suggests that the pathogenic stimulus should be associated with only one disease. This is not a particularly rigorous criterion as there is much evidence that individual stimuli are capable of causing more than one type of illness. For example, exposure to tobacco smoke can cause lung cancer,[13,14] but it is also causally associated with cancers of the bladder,[18] larynx and oesophagus, and coronary artery disease.

4. **Temporality.** Temporality is a particularly important consideration for diseases of long latency. It is essential that exposure to the pathogen occurred before the onset of the disease. Investigators must be sure that an illness observed in a particular environmental setting is caused by that environment rather than by sick people migrating into that environment.

5. **Biological gradient.** A dose–response gradient in the epidemiological findings adds greatly to the postulated causal association. Smoking and lung cancer show a very strong dose–response curve. The greater the number of cigarettes smoked the higher the relative risk of lung cancer (Figure 5.2).

   Dose-response is not always linear. Thus, a lack of dose–response does not confirm absence of causality, but its presence adds greatly to the strength of the cause and effect hypothesis.

6. **Plausibility.** The concept of plausibility, which asks that the postulated cause should be biologically plausible, is excellent in theory. However, in practice because plausibility is dependent upon the state of contemporary knowledge, it should not be applied too vigorously.

7. **Coherence.** The concept of coherence is more rigorous than plausibility

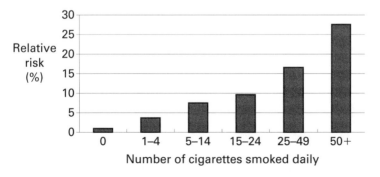

Figure 5.2. Relative risk for lung cancer in smokers and non-smokers

as it suggests that the interpretation of the cause and effect hypothesis should not seriously conflict with the known facts about the natural history and biology of the disease.

8. **Experimental evidence.** Is there evidence that a similar disease can be produced in experimental animals by the same stimulus? The problem with this is that animals do not always respond to a stimulus in the same way as man. For example, had penicillin been tested on guinea pigs rather than mice it would never have been used for humans, because guinea pigs are extremely sensitive to penicillin.[19]

CHOICE OF CONTROL DISEASE

There are some basic principles which must be considered when selecting the control population. Because the incidence of disease varies with age, sex and social class, the control population should have similar demographic characteristics to those of the study population. It is sometimes useful to compare the distribution of the adverse health outcome with a control disease. The purpose of this is to compare the spatial distribution of the adverse health outcome with that of a control disease. For this technique to work it is essential that the underlying age, sex and social class distributions are the same for both the control disease and postulated adverse health outcome. Also, the control disease should have no known association with the postulated pollutant.

CHOICE OF CONTROL POPULATION

Baseline data about health outcomes in communities are not routinely collected. To determine whether or not there might be a health concern about living in a certain neighbourhood it is necessary to compare the health outcomes in the 'problem' environment with that of a control community. The choice of the control community is very important. It must reflect the demographic characteristics of the study population such as age, sex and social class. But, it must not have any sources of pollution which may adversely affect its residents. This is not always easy to determine. Obvious sources of potential pollution are easy to identify: chimneys belching out black acrid smoke; factories involved in known hazardous productions such as chemicals and oils; and landfill dumps which may or may not attract fly dumping. However, there are many industries which may not be thought of as polluters on first inspection but which, through lapses in maintenance or inadequate management, are seriously polluting the environment. When selecting a control community it is essential that the community is visited and scrutinized thoroughly for any potential sources of pollution.

In some instances the expected difference in health will be small between the control and the study community. In such situations it is advisable to investigate more than one control community. The smaller the anticipated difference in health between the communities, the greater the need for more than one control community.

It is sometimes difficult to identify a suitable control population. The characteristics of some populations make them appear unique and thus difficult to match in other communities. One way of overcoming such a problem is to ask each person in the study population to recommend a control for himself or herself.[20] This approach usually ensures that the controls are representative of the study population. It is a particularly valuable approach if it is incorporated within a study design which uses more than one control community.

A POSSIBLE TEMPLATE

The following pages outline one approach to investigating a suspected environmental hazard in a community.

INITIAL RESPONSE: COLLECTING INFORMATION

The first indication of a possible problem often comes from anecdotal reports from the community. If you decide to investigate the reports more

Table 5.2. Initial information collected

• Describe the characteristics of the disease	• Suspected source of exposure
	• Numbers affected
	• Geographical area affected
	• Time period
• Describe the characteristics of the people affected	• Sex
	• Age
	• Residence
	• Occupation
• Search for additional cases	• Determine geographical area
	• Determine appropriate denominator
	• Calculate rates and compare to an appropriate standard population
• Verify diagnosis	• Initially through informal contacts with GPs and hospital staff

fully the initial response should be aimed at elucidating the characteristics of the disease and the population affected.

DEVELOP THE HYPOTHESIS

Many factors will help you to develop a hypothesis such as the clinical features of cases, geographical location of the exposed cases and social conditions of the exposed. The hypothesis is not rigid and may change in light of new information.

DECIDE ON THE DISEASES TO MONITOR

Use a literature search to identify the diseases, a priori, which you would expect to be raised as a result of exposure to the putative pollutant. It is important to cast your net widely in your choice of disease to monitor: (i) because you may have identified a novel association (see Bradford-Hill's criterion of plausibility); or (ii) you may have identified incorrectly the types of pollution in the plume.

DEFINE THE POPULATION AT RISK

It is important to define the population at risk in terms of their demographic characteristics (age, sex, ethnic group, geographical location and occupation). To measure the occurrence of the disease and to compare risks, you need to calculate rates of the disease. This requires knowledge of the number of cases and the total number in the population at risk. Pay attention to susceptible populations—the old, the young and the sick; these groups might be the first affected by pollution. The exposed population must be clearly distinguished from the non-exposed population to avoid dilution of the disease rates.

DESCRIBE THE RATES OF DISEASE

Rates of disease may be calculated for deaths or for illnesses. There are three common measures of mortality: age-specific death rates, standardized mortality ratio, and relative risk. For each method data are needed about the underlying causes of death. For countries and major cities and towns, these data are published in governmental annual statistical publications. Information about the numbers and cause of deaths in smaller communities is available for England and Wales from the Office of National Statistics; for

Scotland from the Information Statistics Division, Common Services Agency; and for Northern Ireland from the Department of Social Security (see Chapter 4).

Only cases of cancer and the notifiable diseases are collected routinely and morbidity rates may be calculated for these diseases. Ad hoc information may be used from other sources such as emergency admissions to hospital, general practitioner consultations, hospital outpatient attendances and sickness absence records.

MAPPING THE DISEASE DISTRIBUTION

Knowledge about the geographical location of disease provides essential information about its cause. Dot maps can clearly identify point sources of pollution and are used routinely in offices of public health personnel to monitor the spread of infectious diseases. They are essential also for describing the relation between a putative pollution source and ill health in a community. Dot maps tend to be limited to small communities, that is one town or village, because of the impossibility of depicting information on large populations clearly. Count maps, adjusted for age and sex, provide summary information about groups of individuals and are used to portray health in larger communities or when information is not available for individuals. Contour mapping is particularly useful when trying to identify populations at risk from exposure. Knowledge about levels of pollution in certain areas, provided by monitoring, can be presented and analysed using contour mapping. The resultant contour map can clearly identify populations at risk from pollution.

ANALYTICAL STAGE

The hypotheses should be clearly stated at the start of the research project. Doing so focuses the study and is more likely to ensure that the study design is appropriate.

The size of the study is vital to the success of your research. The study should be large enough to yield clear answers. The smaller the difference in disease occurrence that you expect to find between the study community and the control community, the larger the sample size needs to be. There are many programmes and publications[21] which enable researchers to choose the appropriate sample size. Unless you are very sure of your approach, it is worth while seeking out the advice of a statistician at a very early stage in the evolution of your research. The key question that you may be asked is the effect size of interest. For instance, if 6% of your control community suffers from a disease and you would be concerned if the rate in the study community was 9%, then the effect size is 3%. In addition, relevant statistical procedures may be suggested, which will quantify the evidence for or against the map hypotheses.

WORKED EXAMPLE

THE ARBROATH MULTIPLE DISEASE STUDY

The remainder of this chapter uses the format of the template previously outlined for describing an investigation about a suspected point source of pollution.

Initial Response/Background

Previous surveys of patterns of environmentally sensitive respiratory disease in central Scotland had demonstrated a high mortality from lung cancer in residential areas of towns downwind of foundries.[22-24] The town of Arbroath in eastern Scotland contained a central industrial area which housed a foundry.

Complaints of dust and fumes in the neighbourhood had been reported during the 1960s and 1970s. At that time, the fumes from the foundry emanated from a hole in the roof of the building. The absence of a fumestack would have exacerbated the tendency of the pollution to accumulate nearby when winds were light or absent. During the late 1970s and throughout the 1980s, the pollution was diminished, first because of an industrial recession and later because pollution control technology had been installed. Thus we collected data for the years 1966–76. The 10-year period allowed also for a reasonable occurrence of disease in the area.

Hypothesis

Due to concerns about the effects of this centrally located foundry on the health status of the surrounding community, it was decided to examine the spatial distribution of mortality arising for a range of diseases in the town area. Specifically the study aimed to test the hypothesis that deaths from bronchitis, gastric, oesophageal and lung cancer would be raised in areas affected by pollution from the foundry.

Selection of Diseases to Monitor

For all residents in the town, information was extracted from the death certificates for the years 1966–76 on age, sex, address, occupation, and the causes of death. Certificates with any mention of lung cancer were used unless the cancers were secondary to a primary cancer in another tissue. The address of each death was plotted on a map. The addresses of deaths with non-respiratory cancers were also extracted from the death certificates and the locations mapped. Two categories of non-malignant disease were selected from the death certificates: ischaemic heart disease where no other significant disease was mentioned and bronchitis. From the list of cases of ischaemic heart disease control deaths were selected which matched with the respiratory cancer deaths by 10-year age-group and by sex, to the closest year of death and to the closest death certificate number if within the same year.

Cancers of the lower body and deaths from ischaemic heart disease were used as control diseases.

Identification of the Population at Risk

The town was divided into four geographical areas by aggregating the enumeration districts of the 1971 census, which were geographically coherent. Area 1 consisted of the residential zones directly to the east and west of the foundry. This area was considered, a priori, to have been potentially at risk from the air pollution because of the prevailing wind directions in Scotland. The remainder of the town was divided into comparison areas 2 (north and south), 3 (west) and 4 (east). There are no particular topographic effects relating to this study.

Rates of Disease

The expected numbers of deaths from respiratory cancer in the four areas were calculated using indirect standardization. The Scottish rates for 1971 provided the standard population. Standardized mortality ratios were calculated for the age-groups 15 and over. The mean standardized mortality ratios for the years 1966–76 of the town's four areas were derived from the values for the observed and expected numbers of deaths within those areas. The statistical significance of the odds ratio of each standardized mortality ratio was calculated.

Mapping the Distribution of Disease

The locations of all cases dying from ischaemic heart disease in 1966, 1971 and 1976 and of bronchitis 1966–76 were mapped. The grid coordinates of these deaths, and of the deaths from respiratory cancer, all non-respiratory cancer, gastric cancer, colorectal cancer, female breast cancer, prostate cancer and cancer of the bladder and kidney were determined. The distributions of these categories of death were illustrated using three-dimensional mapping.[25] The method involves producing surfaces of the local density of cases where elevated areas relate to high density and low areas to low density. The resulting surface maps are produced by an 'optimal' smoothing method (cross-validation).[26]

Results

There were 168 death certificates with the diagnosis of respiratory cancer with addresses within areas 1–4 of Arbroath between 1966 and 1976, and 538 with the diagnosis of other cancers. A cluster of deaths from respiratory cancer was found in area 1, and a smaller cluster in part of area 3. When the SMRs were calculated for the areas (Table 5.3), only area 1 showed a high

Table 5.3. Standardized mortality ratios for lung cancer, non-respiratory cancer and coronary heart disease in the four areas of Arbroath, 1966–76

Areas	OBS	EXP	SMR	95% CI
Respiratory cancer				
1	29	19	153	103 to 220
2	44	47	94	68 to 126
3	36	41	88	62 to 122
4	59	58	101	77 to 130
Non-respiratory cancer				
1	102	56	183	149 to 222
2	145	133	109	92 to 128
3	122	117	104	87 to 125
4	169	159	106	91 to 123
Coronary heart disease				
1	17	19	90	52 to 143
2	43	47	92	66 to 123
3	51	41	125	93 to 164
4	56	58	96	73 to 125

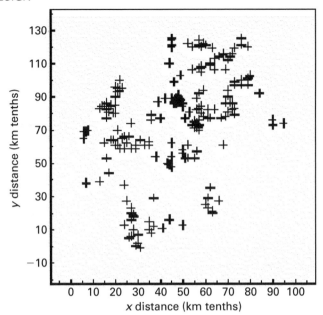

Figure 5.3. Bronchitis case address location map: Arbroath

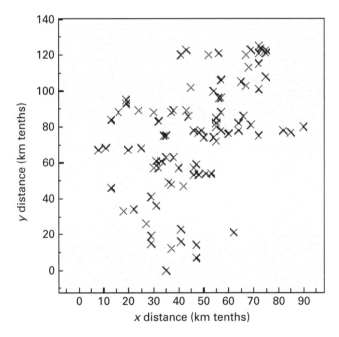

Figure 5.4. Gastric and oesophageal cancer address location map: Arbroath

value. Area 1 contained the highest male age-specific death rates for the age-groups 55–64 and 65–74, and the second highest for the age-group 75+.

Area 1 also contained the highest value for the SMRs for non-respiratory cancer (Table 5.3); the value of 183 was statistically significant. The standardized mortality ratios for the matched controls, who had died of coronary heart disease, did not show significant elevation of the values in area 1 compared to the other areas (Table 5.3).

Figures 5.3 to 5.7 show the spatial distributions of residential locations for deaths from bronchitis, gastric and oesophageal cancer, lung cancer, cancer of the lower body, and ischaemic heart disease.

To act as comparison the spatial distributions of ischaemic heart disease and cancers of the lower body were used as control diseases for bronchitis, gastric and oesophageal cancer, and respiratory cancer. With one control sample we can apply some simple statistical models to assess the relation between the disease location and the foundry location. These models are discussed more fully in Chapter 6. Briefly, we can specify a model for the

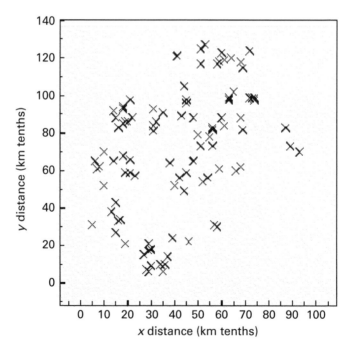

Figure 5.5. Lung cancer address location map: Arbroath

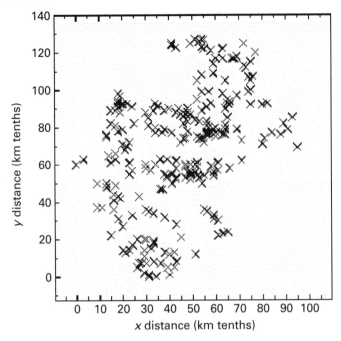

Figure 5.6. Lower body cancers control address location map: Arbroath

excess risk around a source by defining a local density of cases ($\lambda(x)$) at location x, which is a function of the local population at risk (represented by the spatial distribution of the control disease, cancers of the lower body) and a function of exposure variables related to the source location. For our example, the function of exposure variables could be simply based on distance from the source. A simple form of relation is given by $1 + \alpha_1 \exp(-\alpha_2 r(x) + \alpha_3 \log r(x))$ where $r(x)$ is the distance of a case location from the source location. Here the three parameters control the degree of association with the source: α_1 represents the overall association, while α_2 and α_3 represent the degree of evidence related to distance and peak-decline effects (see Chapter 6 for greater detail on these models).

It should be noted that the spatial distribution of the two controls is similar, and this adds weight to the appropriateness of their use in this study. The diseases most likely to show an association with the foundry (respiratory cancer and bronchitis) peak to the southwest and north of the source. Gastric and oesophageal cancers, which were also hypothesized to show an association with the foundry, peak on a northeast–southwest axis. But the

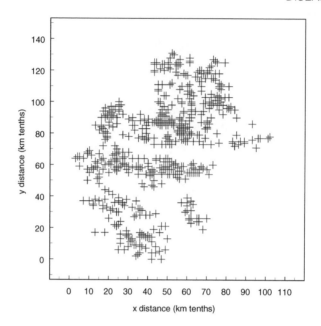

Figure 5.7. Ischaemic heart disease mortality address location map: Arbroath

pronounced peak only occurs to the northeast of the foundry. Thus, while respiratory cancer and bronchitis have similar spatial forms, gastric and oesophageal cancer show different spatial forms.

A complete analysis of these data would consider a possible exploratory analysis of smoothed maps of relative risk (see Chapter 4) and further analysis could be based on tests or statistical modelling of the relation of distance and direction from the source to the case locations. These methods are discussed more fully in Chapter 6.

REFERENCES

1. Lenihan J (1985). *Bonnybridge/Denny Morbidity Review*: Scottish Home and Health Department.
2. Elliott P, Hills M, Beresford J, Kleinschmidt I, Jolley D, Pattenden S *et al.* (1992). Incidence of cancers of the larynx and lung cancer near incinerators of waste solvents and oils in Great Britain. *Lancet* **339**(i): 854–8.
3. Caramaschi F, Del Corno G, Favaretti C, Giambelluca SE, Montesarchio E and

---

SUMMARY

1. The purpose of any study must determine the study design. The issues important in disease mapping or ecological analysis are different from those found in clustering studies.
2. The analysis of putative sources of hazard has particular issues relating to study design. For instance, prevailing wind direction, umbrella effect, identification of diseases to monitor, choice of years to study, and data validation and quality.
3. Choice of study area is extremely important in ecological and cluster studies. For the study of putative hazards a balance between large-scale and small-scale study regions must be made.
4. The choice of time period is very important where latency periods are encountered (e.g. with cancers). The choice of a suitable aggregation level for a particular study is also important.
5. Bradford Hill's criteria for causation provide a good (although potentially fallible) framework to guide your thinking and interpretation of data.

Fara GM (1981). Chloracne following environmental contamination by TCDD in Seveso, Italy. *International Journal of Epidemiology* **10**: 135–43.
4. Bonaccorsi A, Fanelli R and Tognoni G (1978). In the wake of Seveso. *Ambio* **7**(5–6): 234–9.
5. Lloyd OL and Barclay R (1979). A short latency period for respiratory cancer in a 'susceptible' population. *Community Medicine* **1**: 210–20.
6. Goyer RA (1986). Toxic effects of metals. In: Klaassen CD and Doull J (eds). Casarett and Doull's Toxicology: The Basic Science of Poisons, 3rd edn. New York: Macmillan, 582–635.
7. Kimborough R, Buckley J and Fishbein L (1978). Animal toxicology. *Environmental Health Perspectives* **24**: 173–85.
8. McConnell E (1980). Acute and chronic toxicity, carcinogenesis, reproduction, teratogenesis and mutagenesis in animals. *Topics in Environmental Health* **4**: 109–50.
9. Dorozynski A (1994). Chernobyl damaged health, says study. *British Medical Journal* **309**(12 Nov): 1321.
10. Trout KS (1981). How to read clinical journals: IV To determine etiology or causation. *CMA Journal* **124**: 985–90.
11. Bradford Hill A (1965). The environment and disease: association or causation? *Proceedings of the Royal Society of Medicine: Section of Occupational Medicine*.

12. Kimborough RD, Mahaffey KR, Grandjean P, Sandoe S-T and Rutstein DD (1989). *Clinical Effects of Environmental Chemicals.* New York: Hemisphere Publishing Corporation.
13. Doll R and Bradford Hill A (1950). Smoking and carcinoma of the lung. *British Medical Journal* **ii**: 739–48.
14. Wynder EL and Graham EA (1950). Tobacco smoking as a possible etiologic factor in bronchiogenic carcinoma. *The Journal of the American Medical Association* **143**(4): 329–36.
15. Doll R and Hill A (1954). The mortality of doctors in relation to their smoking habits. *British Medical Journal* **i**: 1451–5.
16. Hammond EC and Horn D (1954). The realtionship between human smoking habits and death rates. *Journal of the American Medical Association* **155**: 1316–28.
17. Doll R, Peto R, Wheatley K, Gray R and Sutherland I (1994). Mortality in relation to smoking: 40 years' observations on male British doctors. *British Medical Journal* **309**: 901–11.
18. Notani PN, Shah P, Jayant K and Balakrishnan V (1993). Occupation and cancers of the lung and bladder: A case control study in Bombay. *International Journal of Epidemiology* **22**(2): 185–91.
19. Wilson D (1976). *Pencillin in perspective.* London: Faber and Faber.
20. Schlesselman JJ (1982). *Case Control Studies. Design, Control, Analysis.* Oxford: Oxford University Press, pp. 76–80.
21. Florey CdV (1993). Sample size for beginners. *British Medical Journal* **306**: 1181–4.
22. Lloyd OL, Williams FLR and Gailey FAY (1985). Is the Armadale epidemic over? Air pollution and mortality from lung cancer and other disease, 1961–1982. *British Journal of Industrial Medicine* **42**: 815–23.
23. Lloyd OL, Barclay R and Lloyd MM (1985). Lung cancer and other health problems in a Scottish industrial town. *Ambio* **14**: 322–8.
24. Lloyd OL, Smith G, Lloyd MM AND Gailey F (1985). Raised mortality from lung cancer and high sex ratios of births associated with industrial pollution. *British Journal of Industrial Medicine* **42**: 475–80.
25. Williams FL, Lawson AB and Lloyd OL (1992). Low sex ratios of births in areas at risk from air pollution from incinerators, as shown by geographical analysis and 3-dimensional mapping. *International Journal of Epidemcology* **21**(2): 311–9.
26. Hastie TJ and Tibshirani RJ (1990). *Generalized Additive Models.* London: Chapman & Hall.
27. Bertazzi PA et al. (1989). Mortality in an area contaminated by TCDD following an industrial incident. *La Medicina del Lavoro* **80**: 316–29.

6

Advanced Methods

SMOOTHING OF RATES AND DENSITY ESTIMATION

In previous chapters, some simple methods were discussed for use in the production of disease maps. These methods can be implemented easily and are in widespread use for the production of disease atlases and for health planning.[1] However, there are some disadvantages in the use of maps of SMRs or SMDs which have led to the development of more sophisticated methods of disease mapping.

The mapping of ratios or differences, as described in Chapter 4, can contain *artefacts* which affect interpretation. These artefacts might be related to the nature of the measures used (for example ratios or differences) and might also be due to extra variation in the small area data. For example, it is often the aim of a mapping study to assess the *excess* of disease beyond that given by the expected number for any given region. The SMR measures this by comparing observed to expected numbers in the form of a ratio. Values of the SMR greater that 1 may suggest excess risk. However, SMRs can yield risk estimates with wide variability, due to *small* expected rates (e.g. a count of one case in a tract with expectation 0.1, gives an SMR of 10, or when the expectation is 0 then the SMR is infinite). These types of artefact are sometimes avoided by simple transformations of the measure. For example, it is possible to add small constants to the numerator and denominator of an SMR, i.e.

$$\frac{n_i + a}{e_i + b}.$$

This form of transformation makes some allowance for the artefacts inherent in ratios, but does not make any allowance for extra variation in the data. Note also that the use of differences (e.g. SMDs) does not suffer from such severe artefacts as SMRs. SMRs have a direct interpretation as a measure of multiplicative increase in risk, whereas the SMD is a measure of additive risk. Figures 6.1, 6.2 and 6.3 display the effect of changes to the *a* and *b* parameters applied to the Falkirk risk map (Figure 6.1). Figure 6.1 is the SMR map, while Figure 6.2 shows the map of the risks with *a = 0.5*, *b = 0.5*. Figure 6.3 displays the relative risk map for *a = 2.0*, *b = 0.5*. All maps are displayed on the same five class scale (0.0–0.499, 0.5–0.999, 1.0–1.499, 1.5–1.999, 2.0–3.0). The effect of a large value of *a* is to increase the overall risk, while the small values of *a* and *b* lead to changes

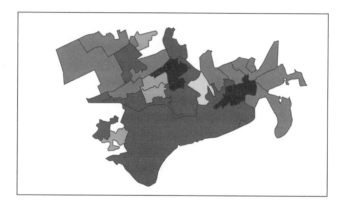

Figure 6.1. Falkirk SMR map

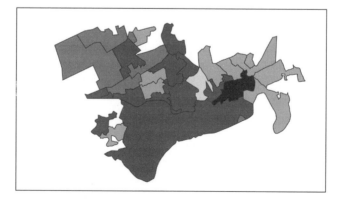

Figure 6.2. Falkirk transformed map: 0.5, 0.5

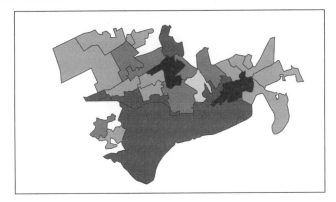

Figure 6.3. Falkirk transformed map : 2.0, 0.5

of high risk area designation (assuming risks greater than two are used as a guide to high risk areas).

The effect of such different transformations should be carefully evaluated as considerable interpretational differences could arise depending on the transformation used. The use of constants a and b has a justification based on a model which assumes that the risk in areas is a random variable (i.e. has extra variation) and it is possible to compute appropriate values of these constants from any data set. The example above is cited simply to illustrate the effects of varying such constants.

Extra variation in disease data can arise from a variety of causes. In the simplest case, it may be that there are many underlying geographical gradients of the aetiological factors for the disease in question that the map does not incorporate. If such gradients exist then the resulting map will contain their imprint. As these effects are not incorporated in the simple measures, discussed above, it can be useful to try to make some allowance for their effect in the analysis. The aggregate effect of such underlying aetiological variables may not be measurable precisely but will be evident from extra variation in the data. This extra variation can take different forms and can be accommodated.

Extra variation leads to increased differences between estimates or measures at different locations. Hence any set of SMRs or SMDs can display such increased differences. This type of extra variation can be accommodated in the map construction by using a *smoothing* method which reduces the differences between peaks and troughs in the disease distribution.

For the situation where residential addresses of cases are used, then the use of *density estimation* to calculate a local rate/intensity of disease is itself a form of smoothing operation, which converts the exact locations into a local density. Density estimation is a statistical method which converts the locations of data into a continuous surface representing the local density of the locations. Such smoothing can be achieved by computing the local (kernel) estimate of the measure of interest (e.g. the SMR or the local case density). These methods provide a weighted averaging of the data across all the data at the locations specified. Hence a kernel estimate of the SMR in one region would involve a weighted average of SMRs across the study region. The weights would be based on a decreasing function of distance from the region of interest to the other regions. A range of smoothing methods can be based on this method. In addition, it is possible to apply this method to control locations and form the ratio of case density to control density to assess any excess risk in areas of the map.

If either approach is applied to SMRs or case/control maps, in both cases the method includes a constant which controls the degree of smoothness of the resulting surface, and a variety of methods can be used to find the best value for this constant. Figure 6.4 shows a kernel smoothed SMR map of

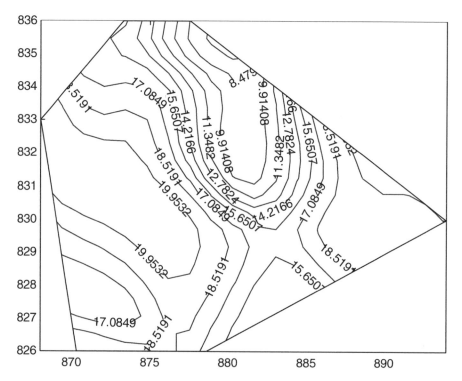

Figure 6.4. Falkirk kernel smoothed SMR map (contours expressed as SMR × 10)

the Falkirk data. The effect of smoothing is to reduce variation across the map to produce a smoothly varying surface. This map now displays the continuous variation on relative risk and has removed peaks and troughs in the data. What remains is the clear areas in the west and east of the map of high risk and the trough in the northern region. The boundaries of the map are simplified from the original map (Figure 6.1). Further interpretation could be aided by superimposition of the tract boundary map.

ECOLOGICAL ANALYSIS

Ecological analysis is closely associated with disease mapping. The focus of ecological studies is the relationship between measured covariables and geographical disease distribution. Usually, hypotheses concerning aetiological factors and disease risk are to be examined. The aetiological relationship may have a spatial expression, because spatial distribution can help to examine a wide variety of aetiological conditions sometimes not available when conventional cohort studies are used. This may be because cohort studies can be prone to censoring of information. An early ecological study involving spatial analysis was the British Regional Heart Study.[2] In that work, disease case numbers in regions were related to regionally averaged explanatory variables, via a regression model including spatial autocorrelation. The regression model allowed for the correlation between neighbouring sites in the study. Additionally, ecological studies are often associated with changes in the resolution level of the measurements made on covariables. For example, numerator data may be available by residential address but the expected death rates may be derived only from census tracts. In this situation, the expected deaths are available at a lower level of resolution than the cases. The *ecological* and *atomistic* fallacy are two concepts which should be considered when undertaking an ecological study. They affect the main data types used in geographical disease studies, namely area counts and individual event locations. The ecological fallacy arises when an attempt is made to ascribe to individuals the characteristics which have been derived from the properties of groups of population. The atomistic fallacy is the opposite. It arises when an individual's disease experience is used to impute average characteristics for a population group. Both of these problems arise when *different* data units are used in a study of relationships. *Any* regression or correlation exercise usually makes an attempt to assess the relationship between measurements at different resolutions, although in ordinary regression the observations are usually made on the same subject.

Ecological and atomistic fallacies have several effects on statistical methods. First, care must be taken in the interpretation of the estimated relationships, when the numerator and denominator derive from different data areas or aggregates. Special models may be required to deal specifically with such situations. The analysis of putative sources of health hazard is a special case of ecological analysis where a specific small set of explanatory covariables, such as distance, direction, and functions of distance around a putative source, are used to explain the disease distribution. Secondly, the issue of measurement error in covariables should be considered. This can occur when a covariable can only be measured with error or could arise due to the necessity of interpolation of covariables to locations of interest. For instance, deprivation indices are now routinely available for census regions/ areas in the UK. However, these may have associated measurement error due to uncertainty in the population characterization in each area. This error should be incorporated in any study associating deprivation indices and disease distribution. Another common example of such error is found when covariables are only measured at locations other than those of the disease measurement: pollution levels are often measured in networks, and these networks do not usually relate directly to health data measurement units. Usually, the pollution level in the vicinity of individual cases of disease is estimated by *interpolation* of measurements. Interpolation methods are characterized by smoothing operations which include some propagation of error to the site of interest. In a spatial setting, it might be appropriate to use Kriging[3] or, possibly, nonparametric kernel smoothers[3] to provide such interpolation. In general, such propagation of error can be seen as an extra element within a hierarchical Bayesian modelling approach, where different sources of error in an analysis are given a probability distribution and these sources of error form a hierarchy. A number of examples of this approach have been reported.[2] Finally, specific *spatial* concerns can arise in ecological studies.

Edge effects (see Chapter 4) can occur when data external to the study region are not available (censored), and also when the model or estimation method assumed for the data depends on neighbourhoods. If small area relative risks are to be estimated then there could be considerable edge effects (within edge areas at least). If the estimation method required the *local* estimation based on a small neighbourhood of the area in question, then there are two consequences. Firstly, if external tract counts are not available then censoring will occur and bias may result in the edge area relative risk estimate. Secondly, even if external areas are not present, as in an island, the estimation method may require that neighbourhoods be used in the estimation process. In the case of edge areas, these usually have fewer neighbours and this can affect both the bias and variability of edge area estimates.

PUTATIVE SOURCES OF HEALTH HAZARD

The assessment of the impact of sources of pollution on the health status of communities is of considerable academic and public concern. The incidence of many respiratory, skin and genetic diseases is thought to be related to environmental pollution.[4-9] Any localized source of such pollution could give rise to changes in the incidence of such diseases in the adjoining community. In recent years, there has been growing interest in the development of statistical methods[9] for use in the detection of patterns of health events associated with pollution sources. In this chapter, we consider the statistical methodology for the assessment of putative health effects of sources of air pollution. We consider inference and modelling problems and concentrate primarily on the generic problem of the statistical analysis of observed point patterns of case events or area counts, rather than specific features of a particular disease or outcome.

A number of studies utilize data based on the spatial distribution of disease to assess the strength of association with exposure to a pollution source. Raised incidence near the source, or a directional alignment related to a dominant wind direction may provide evidence of such a link. The aim of any analysis of such data is to assess the effect of specific spatial variables rather than general spatial statistical modelling. That is, the researcher is interested in detecting patterns of events near (or exposed to) the focus and less concerned about aggregation of events in other locations. The former type of analysis has been named 'focused clustering'. To date, many pollution-source studies have concentrated on incidence of a single disease (e.g. childhood leukaemia around nuclear power stations or respiratory cancers around waste-product incinerators).[6-10]

The types of data observed could vary from residential addresses of cases to counts of disease (mortality or morbidity) within census areas or other arbitrary spatial regions. The two different data types lead to different modelling approaches. Spatial point process models are appropriate for individual-location data.[4] In the case of summary data, one may use the property that numbers in disjoint regions follow an independent Poisson model and typically log-linear models and related tests are used to analyse such data. The effects of pollution sources are measured often over large geographic areas containing heterogeneous population densities. As a result, the intensity of the underlying point process of cases is heterogeneous. The primary inferential problems arising in putative-source studies are *a posteriori* analyses and multiple comparisons. The well-known problem of *a posteriori* analysis arises when prior knowledge of reported disease occurrence near a putative source leads an investigator to carry out statistical tests or to fit models to data to 'confirm' the evidence. Essentially, this problem may give rise to bias in data collection due to prior knowledge of an apparent effect.

Both Hills and Alexander[1] and Gardner,[7] noted that hypothesis tests and study-region definition could be biased using such an approach (see also [2,3,6]). However, if a study *region* is noted, a priori, to be of interest because it includes a putative pollution source, one does not suffer from the problems associated with *a posteriori* study designs as knowledge of the spatial distribution of disease could not influence the choice of region. The multiple-comparison problem can arise due to the possibility that a multiple of tests may be performed, for multiple diseases or at multiple sites, and this may alter the error rate for the tests. This has been addressed in several ways. Bonferonni's inequality may be used to adjust critical regions for multiple comparisons but the conservative nature of such an adjustment can lead to insensitivity in individual tests. Cumulative *p*-value plotting can be used to assess the number of diseases yielding evidence of association with a particular source. This involves the cumulation of test *p* values across the tests used and comparison of this quantity with a specified sampling distribution.

MODELS FOR INDIVIDUAL EVENTS

In this section, we consider a variety of modelling approaches which may be used when data are recorded as a dot map of disease events. Define A to be a study region.

In analysing events around a pollution source, one usually defines a fixed window or geographical region, A, and all events that occur within this region within a particular time period are recorded (mapped). Thus, the total distribution of events within A is modelled. In the analysis of case events around pollution sources, the long-range or trend components of variation are often of primary concern. These components describe the variation in disease over long distances. The models most appropriate to such situations are point process models, known as heterogeneous Poisson point process models.[6] These models have as their basic component, a function which describes the local density of cases (points) on the map. This function is called the first-order intensity. The function is usually defined as $\lambda(x)$, where x is the location. This function is defined to include components describing the trend or long-range variation in the density of cases.

Event locations usually represent residential addresses of cases and take place within a heterogeneous population that varies both in spatial density and in susceptibility to disease. It is possible to include within the specification of $\lambda(x)$, a function which describes this spatial variation in the population at risk.

This intensity may be parameterized as:

$$\lambda(x) = g(x).f(x, \theta)$$

where $g(x)$ is a function of the population and $f(x, \theta)$ is a parameterized function of risk relative to the location of the pollution source. The focus of interest for assessing associations between events and the source, is inference regarding parameters in $f(x, \theta)$, treating $g(x)$ as a nuisance function.

If we observe m cases within A, then the likelihood conditional on m, is (bar a constant):

$$L = \prod_{i=1}^{m} \lambda(x_i).\exp\left\{ -\int_A \lambda(u)du \right\}$$

The set of x_is are the locations of the cases of disease on the map.

Here, parameters in $f(x, \theta)$ and $g(x\}$ must be estimated. It has been proposed to estimate $g(x)$ from the 'at risk' population, and then to substitute this estimate into the likelihood before estimation of other parameters. The method of estimating $g(x)$ is of some concern both from an epidemiological viewpoint and from the stance of statistical inference. Estimation of $g(x)$ is equivalent to the estimation of the 'denominator' in conventional studies using standardised mortality ratios (SMRs). That is, the population at risk and its geographical variation must be accounted for accurately in the estimation of $g(x)$.

In the study of counts of disease within small geographical areas, often the denominator of the SMR is estimated from the rates of disease in a standard population. For case event data, it is also possible to use expected rates to estimate $g(x)$. However, these rates are often only available at an aggregated geographical level. This means that the estimated $g(x)$ will represent a smoothed average of the 'expected' disease risk over the study area.

An alternative approach is to estimate $g(x)$ from a 'control' disease. Essentially, this approach involves using the geographical distribution of another disease as a surrogate for the geographical distribution of the population at risk. The choice of such a disease is of considerable importance. The disease must reflect closely the population variation of the disease of interest but must also be unaffected by the potential health hazard of interest. In the case of putative health hazards, the case disease could be sensitive to, say, air pollution, so the control disease should be matched to the case disease's risk structure but unaffected by air pollution. An example of such a situation would be the study of the incidence of respiratory disease around a waste incinerator. The control disease should be matched to the age and sex structure of the respiratory disease. Lloyd[5] gives an example where respiratory cancer was used as the case disease while coronary heart disease was used as the control disease, and the geographical distributions of these diseases were compared within the study region. There may be considerable epidemiological debate about which controls should be used in any study, given the need to control the matching of the diseases.

Problems of statistical inference arise when $g(x)$ is estimated as a function and then apparently regarded as constant in subsequent inference concerning $\lambda(x)$.[6,8] Essentially, this procedure ignores the sampling variation in the estimate of $g(x)$. As an alternative, it has been proposed[8] to avoid estimation of $g(x)$ by regarding the control locations and case locations as a set of labels whose binary value is determined by a position-dependent probability. That is, the total set of cases and controls are examined and case locations are given a 1 and control locations a 0. It is then possible to define a probability of a case label (1) at location x, say. This model avoids the use of $g(x)$ and hence avoids the inferential problems mentioned previously. However, this model can *only* be applied when a dot map of a control disease is available and when multiplicative risk is assumed.

The specification of $f(x, \theta)$ is of importance as this determines the relation between the source and the disease of interest. This is often termed *exposure* modelling, as this component determines the type of exposure the researcher would expect, a priori, to find if there were any link between the disease incidence and the source. A number of possible models can be specified, depending on the effects the researcher wants to examine. First a distance decline function, describing the reduction in risk with distance from the source, may be included:

$$f(x, \theta) = 1 + \exp(-\alpha r)$$

where r is the distance of location x from the source. This model includes an additive link between the $g(x)$ function and the excess risk due to the source, thereby preserving the background risk at distance (i.e. when r is large, $f(x, \theta) = 1$). In addition to this simple distance decline model it is possible to add effects describing direction and also a peaked effect with distance from the source. For example:

$$f(x, \theta) = 1 + \exp(\alpha_1 \ln r - \alpha_2 r)$$

includes a peaked component over distance, while

$$f(x, \theta) = 1 + \exp(\alpha_1 \ln r - \alpha_2 r + \cos(\theta) + \sin(\theta))$$

includes also components which measure the directional preference of the cases around the source.

It is possible that population or environmental heterogeneity may be unobserved in the data set (i.e. there may be factors not included in the analysis which affect the risk). This could be because either the population background hazard is not directly available or the disease displays a tendency to cluster (perhaps due to unmeasured covariates). The heterogeneity could be spatially correlated, or it could lack correlation in which case it could be regarded as a type of 'overdispersion' or extra variation.

Such unobserved heterogeneity may be included within the framework of conventional models as a random effect. These effects can be incorporated in any analysis by using Bayesian methods (see[9] and Chapters 1 and 2). The detail of such advanced modelling approaches is beyond the scope of this book however.

ESTIMATION

The parameters of the point process models discussed previously, can be estimated by maximum likelihood, if an estimate of $g(x)$ is available.[3,6,8] It is possible to use standard statistical packages such as GLIM or S-Plus for such model fitting, if special integration weighting schemes are used.[10]

HYPOTHESIS TESTS

Tests for spatial effects around putative sources of health hazard have been developed. Possible effects of health hazards on surrounding disease incidence could be found in the relation between distance from the putative source and the pollution source of interest. In addition, the direction from the source to the event location may be important in the case of, for example, air pollution. Tests are available which assess distance, directional and other effects around sources. These tests can be performed in statistical software packages (such as GLIM, GENSTAT or S-Plus) if one uses the special weighting schemes. Tests of monotonic radial decline assume that distance acts as a surrogate for exposure. Many proposed tests are based on radial decline models in point data and tract-count data. An example of such a test for case event data is the score test described by Lawson and Williams.[3,10]

A wide variety of spatial effects could arise due to pollution from a fixed source, and overemphasis on radial decline can yield erroneous conclusions. For example, fallout from stack plumes tends to peak at some distance from a source.[3] Hence, a peak-and-decline intensity may be expected.

Figure 6.5 displays a variety of possible exposure types found around a putative source. These graphs describe idealized distance–risk relationships. Type a describes a simple distance decline relation, which is often used alone to describe the expected exposure around a source. Types b and c could also occur around a source if there is a peak in the distance relation (b) or if the disease clustered naturally (c). If type b or c were realized, then simple radial decline tests (or models) will have low power or unnecessarily high variance. Other exposure models have been suggested which involve constant risk in a disc around the source. However, the justification for constant risk on exposure-path or epidemiological grounds seems scant.

The collection of data and spatial modelling of exposure levels should lead to increased power to detect pollution effects. Unobserved heterogeneity may be included as random effects. Alternatively, the heterogeneity may be formulated in terms of nuisance parameters. Lawson and Harrington[11]

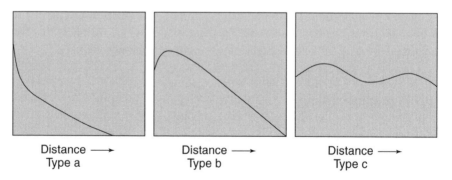

Distance ⟶   Distance ⟶   Distance ⟶
Type a   Type b   Type c

Figure 6.5. Distance–risk relationships

examined Monte Carlo tests, in a putative source setting, when spatial correlation is present and can be estimated as a nuisance effect under the null hypothesis.

MODELS FOR COUNT DATA

For a variety of reasons, data may be available only as numbers within small census regions rather than as precise event locations. As a result, a considerable literature has developed concerning the analysis of such data.[3]

The usual model adopted for the analysis of summary area data around putative pollution hazards, assumes that the numbers in the p regions of interest are independent Poisson random variables with parameters $\{\lambda_i\}$, $i = 1, \ldots, p$. When λ_i is parameterized as a log-linear function, one often treats explanatory variables (in particular exposure or radial distance or direction from a pollution source) as constants for the sub-regions or as occurring at region centres (centroids) only. Such log-linear models can be useful in describing the global characteristics of a spatial pattern. However, the underlying process of events may not support the Poisson distributional assumption. Assessments of such model assumptions could be an important aspect of any study design.[12]

Analysis based on regional summaries is ecological in nature and inference can suffer from the 'ecological fallacy' of attributing effects observed in aggregate to individuals. Extreme rarity of the disease (and therefore large numbers of zero counts) can lead to a bimodal marginal (non-spatial) distribution of counts or invalidate asymptotic sampling distributions.[13] To deal with these situations, it is possible to use tests which are based on simulation (Monte Carlo tests).[3]

The independent Poisson model may be a useful starting point from which to examine effects of pollution sources.[14,15] Often, a log-linear model parameterization is used, with an expected rate value e_i, say, which acts as the contribution of the population of the ith sub-region to the expected number in the ith sub-region. Usually the expected count/number is modelled as

$$\lambda_i = e_i.m\{f\alpha\}$$

Here, the e_i act as a background rate for the ith sub-region. The function $m(.)$ represents a link to spatial and other covariates in the matrix f. Define the polar coordinates of the sub-region centre (centroid) as

$$\{r_i, \theta_i\}$$

relative to the pollution source. Often, the only variable to be included in f is r, the distance from the source. When this is used alone, an additive link such as $m(.) = 1 + \exp(.)$, is appropriate since (for distance decline) the background rate, e_i, is unaltered at great distances. However, directional variables (e.g. $\cos(\theta)$, $\sin(\theta)$, $\sin(\theta)$, etc.), representing preferred direction, can also be useful in detecting directional preference of pollution fallout.

This model may be extended to include unobserved heterogeneity between regions by introducing a prior distribution for the log relative risks $\{\log(\lambda_i)\}$. This could be defined to include spatially uncorrelated or correlated heterogeneity. Bayesian methods are often used in this approach.

ESTIMATION

The parameters of the log-linear model, just described previously, may be estimated via maximum likelihood, through standard Generalized Linear Modelling (GLM) packages, such as GLIM or S-Plus. Using a GLM, the known log of the background hazard for the sub-regions, $\log(e_i)$, $i = 1, \ldots, p$ are treated as 'offsets' (i.e. known constants). A multiplicative (log) link can be directly modelled in this way, while an additive link can be programmed via special procedures. Lawson[15] gives examples of this type of analysis in an application to the analysis of bronchitis mortality around a waste product incinerator.

Log-linear models are appropriate if due care is taken to examine whether model assumptions are met. To avoid the violation of large-sample sampling distributions, use can be made of Monte Carlo tests for goodness-of-fit of the models. The deviance measures the goodness-of-fit of any given model. If a model fits well, then the standardized model residuals should be approximately independently and identically distributed (i.i.d.). One may use autocorrelation tests, again via Monte Carlo, and make any required model adjustments. If such residuals are not available directly, then it is always possible to compare crude model residuals to a simulation of m sets of residuals generated from the fitted model.

Bayesian models for count data can be sampled via Markov chain Monte Carlo (MCMC) methods, and a variety of approximations are also available to provide empirical Bayes estimates. Details of these advanced methods are available in Carlin and Louis.[16]

HYPOTHESIS TESTS

Most of the existing literature on area counts of health effects of pollution sources is based on hypothesis testing.[3,17] Stone[17] first outlined tests specifically designed for summary data around a pollution source. These tests are based on the ratio of observed to expected counts cumulated over distance from a pollution source. The tests are based on the assumption of independent Poisson counts with monotonic distance ordering of the numbers in regions with distance from the source. A number of case studies have been based on these tests.[3]

While Stone's test is based on traditional epidemiological estimates (i.e. SMRs), the test is not uniformly most powerful for detecting a monotonic trend. If such a test exists, it is a score test for particular clustering alternative hypotheses (for example the Lawson–Waller test).[6,15]

The power of a range of such tests has been examined and it was found that all tests had low power against non-monotone or clustered alternatives. Unfortunately, these forms of alternative commonly arise in small-area epidemiological studies. Tests designed to incorporate a peaked effect and where clustering occurs in the background have also been developed.[11,15]

DISEASE CLUSTERING

The analysis of clusters of disease has generated considerable interest within public health. This interest grew during the 1980s, partly due to growing concerns about adverse environmental effects on the health status of populations. In particular, concerns about the influence of nuclear power installations on the health of surrounding populations, have given rise to the development of methods which seek to evaluate clusters of disease.[7,18–32] These clusters are regarded as representing local adverse health risk conditions, possibly ascribable to environmental causes. However, it is also true that for many diseases the geographical incidence of disease will naturally display clustering at some spatial scale, even after the 'at risk' population effects are taken into account.[21] The reasons for such clustering of disease are various. First, it is possible that for some *apparently* non-infectious diseases there may be a viral agent, which could induce clustering. This has been hypothesized for example for childhood leukaemia.[21] Second, other common but so far unknown factors/variables could lead to the apparent clustering. For example, localized pollution sources could produce elevated incidence of disease (for example road junctions could yield high carbon monoxide levels and hence may be hypothesized to lead to elevated respiratory disease incidence). Alternatively, the common treatment of diseases can lead to clustering of disease side effects. The prescription of a drug by a medical practice could lead to elevated incidence of disease within that practice area. Hence, there are many situations where diseases may be found to cluster, even when the aetiology does not suggest this should be observed. Because of this, it is important to be aware of the role of clustering methods, as even when clustering *per se* is not the main focus of interest, it may be important to consider clustering as a background effect and to employ appropriate methods to detect such effects.

DEFINITION OF CLUSTERS AND CLUSTERING

A wide variety of definitions have been suggested[18,21] for the definition of clusters. However, it is convenient here to consider two extreme forms of clustering within which most definitions can be subsumed. First, researchers may not wish to define, a priori, the exact form/extent of clusters to be studied, then a nonparametric definition is often the basis adopted. An example of such a definition for a cluster is given by Knox: 'a geographically bounded group of occurrences of sufficient size and concentration to be unlikely to have occurred by chance'.[18]

Without any assumptions about shape or form of the cluster then the most basic definition would be: *any area within the study region of significant elevated risk*. This definition is often referred to as *hot spot* clustering. This is a simpler form of Knox's definition but summarizes the essential ingredients. In essence any area of elevated risk, regardless of shape or extent, could qualify as a cluster, provided the area meets some statistical criteria. It is not usual to regard areas of significantly low risk as of interest, although these may have some importance in studies of the aetiology of a particular disease. Secondly, at the other extreme, we can define a parametric cluster form: *the study region has a prespecified cluster structure*. This definition describes a parameterized cluster form which is considered to apply across the whole study region. Usually this implies some stronger prior form for the cluster and also some region-wide parameters which control cluster form.

Both of the preceding examples of clustering extremes can be modified by modelling approaches which borrow from either form. It is possible to model cluster form parametrically, but also to include a nonparametric component in the cluster estimation part which allows for a variety of cluster shapes across the study region. As implied, these two clustering extremes represent the spectrum of modelling from nonparametric to parametric forms; associated with these forms are appropriate statistical models and estimation procedures. Any model or test relating to general clustering will assess some overall/global aspect of the clustering tendency of the disease of interest. This could be summarized by a model parameter (such as an autocorrelation parameter in an appropriate model) or by a test which assesses the aggregation of cases of disease. Many general clustering methods[24–28] are available which assess whether a study region has clustering within it. These methods can be regarded as *non-specific* in that they do not seek to estimate the spatial locations of clusters, but simply to assess whether clustering is apparent in the study region. Any method which seeks to assess the locations of clusters (i.e. *where* the clusters are located) is defined to be *specific*.

A second class of clustering methods are termed *focused* and *nonfocused*. These are specific methods for examining one or more clusters and their locational structure. Focused clustering is defined as the study of clusters where the location and number of the clusters is predefined. In that case, only the extent of clustering around the predefined locations is to be modelled. Examples of this approach mainly come from studies of putative sources of health hazard, for example the analysis of disease incidence around prespecified *foci* which are thought to be sources of health hazard. Recent studies include: nuclear power installations,[7] waste dumps,[21] incinerators,[15] harbours,[21] road intersections[21] or steel foundries.[10] In this section we consider only the non-focused form of clustering as focused clustering is dealt with in the section on putative sources of hazard.

Within any analysis of geographically distributed health data, it is important to consider the structure of hypotheses which could include cluster components. Many examples of published analyses within the areas of disease mapping using focused clustering consider the null hypothesis that the observed disease incidence arises only from the underlying *at risk* population distribution. The assumption is made that, once this population is accurately estimated, then it is possible to assess any differences between the observed disease incidence and that expected to have arisen from the background population. However, if the disease of interest naturally clusters (beyond that explained by the estimated at risk background), then this form of clustering should be included also within the null hypothesis. As this form of clustering often represents unobserved covariates or confounding variables, it is appropriate to include this as heterogeneity. This can be achieved in many cases via the inclusion of random effects in the analysis.

Such random effects are often *non-specific* in that they do not attempt to model the exact form of clusters but seek to mimic the effect of clustering in the expected incidence of the disease. The correlated and uncorrelated heterogeneity first described by Clayton and Kaldor,[19] and Besag et al.[20] come under this category. If clustering of disease incidence is to be studied under the alternative hypothesis, then not only would heterogeneity be needed under the null hypothesis, but some form of cluster structure must be estimable under the alternative hypothesis as well. In a disease mapping context, a residual can be computed after fitting a model with different types of heterogeneity.[20] This residual could contain uncorrelated error, trend or cluster structure depending on the application. Such a residual could provide a simple nonparametric approach for the exploration of cluster form in some cases. One disadvantage of the use of the non-specific random effects, is that they do not exactly match the usual form of cluster variation in geographical studies. In rare diseases, at least, clusters usually occur as isolated areas of elevated intensity separated by relatively large areas of low intensity. In that case, the use of a log transformed Gaussian random effect model fitted to the whole region, as often advocated, will not closely mimic the disease clustering tendency.

MODELLING ISSUES

The development of models for clusters and clustering has seen greater development in some areas than in others. It is straightforward to formulate a non-specific Bayesian model for case events or area summaries which includes heterogeneity. However, specific models are less often reported. It is possible to formulate specific clustering models for the case event and area summary situation. If it is assumed that the intensity of case events, at a location is $\lambda(x)$, then by specifying a dependence in this intensity on the locations of cluster centres, it is possible to proceed. For example:

$$\lambda(x) = g(x). \sum_{j=1}^{k} h(x - y_i)$$

describes the intensity of events around k centres located at $\{y_j\}$, $j = 1, \ldots, k$. The distribution of events around a centre is defined by a cluster distribution function $h(.)$. Conditional on the cluster centres, a likelihood can be specified. It is possible to formulate this problem as a Bayesian sampling problem, with a mixture of components of unknown number. This type of problem is well suited to iterative estimation methods called Markov chain Monte Carlo (MCMC) methods. The approach can be applied to count data also.[21]

HYPOTHESIS TESTS FOR CLUSTERING

The literature of spatial epidemiology has developed considerably in the area of hypothesis testing and, more specifically, in the sphere of hypothesis testing for clusters. Very early developments in this area arose from the application of statistical tests to spatio-temporal clustering, a particularly strong indicator of the importance of a spatial clustering phenomenon. Early seminal work[22,23] in the field of space–time cluster testing, predates most of the development of spatial cluster testing. As described previously, distinction should be made between tests for general (non-specific) clustering, which assess the overall clustering pattern of the disease, and the specific clustering tests where cluster locations are estimated. For case events, a few tests have been developed for non-specific clustering. Cuzick and Edwards[24] developed a test which is based on a distribution of cases and a sample of a control disease. Functions of the distance between case locations and k 'nearest' cases, were proposed as test statistics (as opposed to controls). The null hypothesis is tested against clustered alternatives. Diggle and Chetwynd[25] extended point process model descriptive measures to the case where a population background is present. Their method uses a complete control disease distribution and also provides a measure of scale of clustering. Neither of these methods allows for the incorporation of trend which may be present in many examples. Anderson and Titterington[26] have proposed the use of a simple integrated squared distance statistic for cluster assessment. This is closely related to the analysis of density ratios in exploratory analysis, and could be regarded as a type of nonparametric assessment of clustering. The advantage of this approach is that the assessment is not tied to a specific cluster model but detects departures from background. The major disadvantage, shared with all such statistics and tests, is its low power against specific forms of clustering.

Other simple forms of global test can be proposed where density estimates of cases are compared to density estimates of case events simulated from the control background. These could provide confidence intervals at the case locations as well as global tests. There appears to have been little development of tests which detect uncorrelated heterogeneity in the intensity of the case process as a form of spatial clustering. It is unclear what aetiological difference would be inferred when uncorrelated rather than correlated forms of heterogeneity were found. The general tests for overall clustering so far proposed, suffer from the problem that often underlying unobserved heterogeneities are common in such data and the tests do not provide mechanisms for the incorporation of such effects. For example, if spatial trend were present in the case events then this effect could be confounded with cluster effects. One solution to this is to adopt a full clustering model, which can be expanded easily to include such effects as trend and heterogeneity, and to test for inclusion of effects within iterative algorithms.

General clustering tests for area summaries, so far developed, can be classified into tests for correlated heterogeneity and tests for uncorrelated heterogeneity. The latter tests are not spatial in origin but are included here for completeness. In the case of correlated heterogeneity, Whittemore et al.[27] developed a test statistic which compared observed counts and expected counts for all tracts weighted by a covariance matrix. This test was found to have reduced power in some situations. Subsequently, a modified general class of tests for general and focused clustering was developed.[28] An alternative procedure based on Moran's I statistic, modified to allow tract-specific expected rates, has also been proposed. All of these tests make approximating assumptions (for instance, that counts are independently Poisson distributed with constant expectation within each area), and are unlikely, therefore, to perform well against specific clustering forms. Also they assume that clusters yield a total increase in divergence between count and expectation, while other forms of process could yield equivalent degrees of divergence and hence this could lead to misinterpretation. Some use has been made of tests for uncorrelated heterogeneity to assess cluster-ing of tract counts. The Euroclus project[29] has invested considerable effort in testing for such heterogeneity across European states using the Potthoff–Whittinghill test and score tests for Poisson versus negative binomial distributions for the marginal count distribution. But these tests are approx-imate, in that they assume constant within region expected rate, and they may suffer from considerable interpretational problems when, a priori, there is likely to be some non-specific heterogeneity in small-area data. In addition evidence from the Euroclus project suggests that these tests per-form poorly for certain important forms of non-Poisson alternatives within the negative binomial family. In addition, at least for rare diseases, it is easily possible that the marginal count distribution would not follow a negative binomial distribution and could even display multimodality.

Specific cluster tests address the issue of the location of clusters. These tests produce results in the form of locational probabilities or significances associated with specific groups of counts or cases. Oppenshaw *et al.*[30] first developed a general method which allowed the assessment of the location of clusters of cases within large disease maps. The method was based on repeated testing of counts of disease within circular regions of different sizes. Whenever a circle contains a significant excess of cases it is drawn on the map. After a large number of iterations, the resulting map can contain areas where a concentration of overlapping circles suggests localized excesses of a disease. The statistical foundation of this method has been criticized and an improvement to the method was proposed.[31] Their method involves accumulating events (either cases or counts) around individual event locations. These could be cases or areas. Accumulation proceeds up to a fixed number of events or areas k. The number k is fixed in advance. The method can be carried out for a range of k values. While the local alternative for this test is increased intensity, there appears to be no specific clustering process under the alternative and in that sense the test procedure is nonparametric, except that a monotone cluster distance distribution is implicit. One advantage of the test is that it can be applied to focused clusters, while a disadvantage is that an arbitrary choice of k must be made and the results of the test must depend on this choice.

An alternative statistic has been proposed,[32] which employs a likelihood ratio test for the comparison of an overall binomial likelihood for the study region for number of cases out of a total population (the null hypothesis), to a likelihood which has different binomial components depending on being inside or outside a circular zone of defined size. The test can be applied to both case events and area counts. The advantage of the test is that it examines a potentially infinite range of zone sizes and does rely on a formal model of null and alternative hypotheses. However, some limitations of the method relate to the use of circular regions which tends to emphasize *circular* clusters (as does the Openshaw test), and the choice of crude population as the expression of the background 'at risk' structure.

It is also possible to apply two extreme forms of test for *either* a nonparametric (hot spot) cluster-specific test or a fully parametric form. First, if we assume that n_i and e_i are the count and expected count in the ith sub-region respectively, and we can compare $n_i - e_i$ with $n_{ij}^* - e_i$ for each tract, where n_{ij}^*, $j = 1, \ldots, 99$ are simulated counts for each tract based on the given expectation for that tract. If any tract count exceeds the critical level within the rankings of the simulated residuals then we accept the tract as 'significant'. The resulting map of 'significant' tracts displays clusters of different forms. In the case event situation, comparison of $\hat{\lambda}_i^* - \hat{\lambda}_i$ where $\hat{\lambda}_i^*$

is a density estimate based on the case events only and $\hat{\lambda}_i$ is a density estimate based on the controls only (assuming a control distribution is available) can be made.

This could be compared to a set of events simulated from the density estimate of the controls and their density estimates. At the other extreme, it is possible to test for specific cluster locations via the assumption of a cluster sum term in either the intensity of case events or, in the case of tract counts, the specification of the expected rate in each tract. As the cluster locations and number of locations are random quantities, it would be necessary to employ either approximations which involve fixed cluster numbers or to include testing within iterative algorithms (such as Markov chain Monte Carlo).

SUMMARY

1. Smoothing of disease maps can be important due to artefacts which arise from the method used to estimate the mapped data.
2. Ecological analysis is closely related to disease mapping but has as its focus the relation between covariables and mapped incidence at an aggregate level. It involves estimating average relations and issues relating to inference possible from aggregate relations arise.
3. An important area of concern, particularly as it arises in a routine public health context, is the analysis of putative health hazards. Exposure modelling around putative sources is an important issue. A variety of methods have been developed to model such situations, and a range of hypothesis tests have been developed.
4. Disease clustering is an important issue within public health. It is possible to use hypothesis testing procedures to assess global as well as specific clustering. It is also possible to use advanced methods for cluster modelling. The definition of what constitutes a cluster remains unresolved.

REFERENCES

1. Hills M and Alexander F (1989). Statistical methods used in assessing the risk of disease near a source of possible environmental pollution: a review. *Journal of the Royal Statistical Society* **152**: 353–63.

2. Lawson AB and Cressie NAC (1999). Spatial statistical methods in environmental epidemiology. In Rao CR and Sen PK (eds). *Handbook of Statistics: Bio-Environmental and Public Health*, Volume 18. Amsterdam: Elsevier, (*This review covers the whole area of disease mapping and risk assessment and is a good introduction to the statistical issues in the field.*)

3. Lawson AB, Biggeri A and Williams FLR (1999). A review of modelling approaches in health risk assessment around putative sources. In Lawson *et al.* (eds). *Disease Mapping and Risk Assessment for Public Health*. New York: Wiley/WHO.

4. Diggle P (1983). *Statistical Methods for Spatial Point Processes*. London: Academic Press. (*This is a basic introduction to models useful in studying point processes.*)

5. Lloyd O (1982). Mortality in a small industrial town. In: Gardner A (ed.). *Current Approaches to Occupational Health—2*. London: Wright, pp. 283–309.

6. Lawson AB and Waller L (1996). A review of point pattern methods for spatial modelling of events around sources of pollution. *Environmetrics* **7**: 471–88. (*A recent review of statistical methods applicable in putative hazard source analysis.*)

7. Gardner MJ (1989). Review of reported increases of childhood cancer rates in the vicinity of nuclear installations in the UK. *Journal of the Royal Statistical Society* **152**: 307–25.

8. Diggle P and Rowlingson B (1994). A conditional approach to point process modelling of elevated risk. *Journal of the Royal Statistical Society, Series A* **157**: 433–40.

9. Lawson AB, Biggeri A, Boehning D, Lesaffre E, Viel JF and Bertollini R (1999). *Disease Mapping and Risk Assessment for Public Health*. New York: Wiley/WHO. (*This edited book provides a state-of-the-art overview of advanced methods in this area.*)

10. Lawson AB and Williams FLR (1994). Armadale: a case-study in environmental epidemiology. *Journal of the Royal Statistical Society, Series A*. **157**: 285–98. (*This paper demonstrates many of the techniques and issues relating to the analysis of case event data.*)

11. Lawson AB and Harrington NW (1996). The analysis of putative environmental pollution gradients in spatially correlated epidemiological data. *Journal of Applied Statistics* **7**: 471–88.

12. Diggle P (1993). Point process modelling in environmental epidemiology. In: Barnett V and Turkman K (eds). *Statistics in the Environment SPRUCE I*. New York: Wiley.

13. Zelterman D (1987). Goodness of fit tests for large sparse multinomial distributions. *Journal of the American Statistical Association* **82**: 624–9.

14. Bithell J and Stone R (1988). On statistical methods for analysing the

geographical distribution of cancer cases near nuclear installations. *Journal of Epidemiology and Community Health* **43**: 79–85.

15. Lawson AB (1993). On the analysis of mortality events around a prespecified fixed point. *Journal of the Royal Statistical Society A* **156**: 363–77.
16. Carlin BP and Louis TA (1996). *Bayes and Empirical Bayes Methods for Data Analysis*. London: Chapman & Hall.
17. Stone R (1988). Investigations of excess environmental risks around putative sources: statistical problems and a proposed test. *Statistics in Medicine* **7**: 649–60.
18. Knox EG (1989). Detection of clusters. In Elliott P (ed.). *Methodology of Enquiries into Disease Clustering*. London: Small Area Health Statistics Unit.
19. Clayton D and Kaldor J (1987). Empirical Bayes estimates of age-standardised relative risks for use in disease mapping. *Biometrics* **43**: 671–91.
20. Besag J, York J and Mollie A (1991). Bayesian image restoration with two applications in spatial statistics. *Annals of the Institute of Statistical Mathematics* **43**: 1–59.
21. Lawson AB and Kulldorff M (1999). A review of cluster detection methods. In Lawson *et al.* (eds). *Disease Mapping and Risk Assessment for Public Health*. New York: Wiley/WHO. (*This review covers basic ideas in cluster detection.*)
22. Mantel N (1967). The detection of disease clustering and a generalised regression approach. *Cancer Research* **27**: 209–20.
23. Knox EG (1964). The detection of space–time interactions. *Applied Statistics* **13**: 250–9.
24. Cuzick J and Edwards R (1990). Spatial clustering for inhomogeneous populations (with discussion). *Journal of the Royal Statistical Society, Series B* **52**: 73–104.
25. Diggle P and Chetwynd A (1991). Second-order analysis of spatial clustering for inhomogeneous populations. *Biometrics* **47**: 1155–63.
26. Anderson NH and Titterington DM (1997). Some methods for investigating spatial clustering, with epidemiological applications. *Journal of the Royal Statistical Society* **160**: 87–105.
27. Whittemore A, Friend N, Brown B and Holly E (1987). A test to detect clusters of disease. *Biometrika* **74**: 631–5.
28. Tango, T (1995). A class of tests for detecting 'general' and 'focussed' clustering of rare diseases. *Statistics in Medicine* **14**: 2323–34.
29. Alexander F, Wray N, Boyle P, Coebergh JW, Draper G, Bring J, Levi F, Kinney PAM, Michaelis J, Peris-Bonet R, Petridou E, Pukkala E, Storm H, Terracini B and Vatten L (1996). Clustering of childhood leukaemia: a European study in progress. *Journal of Epidemiology and Biostatistics* **1**: 13–24.
30. Oppenshaw S, Charlton M, Wymer C and Craft A (1987). A mark I geographical analysis machine for the automated analysis of point set data sets. *International Journal of Geographical Information Systems* **1**: 335–58.

31. Besag J and Newell J (1991). The detection of clusters in rare diseases. *Journal of the Royal Statistical Society, Series A* **154**: 143–55.
32. Kulldorff M and Nagarwalla N (1995). Spatial disease clusters: detection and inference. *Statistics in Medicine* **14**: 799–810.

7

Public Health Surveillance and Mapping

PROACTIVE AND REACTIVE MONITORING

THE ROLE OF DISEASE MAPPING IN HEALTH BOARDS

Disease mapping can play an important role in monitoring the health of a community. Plotting new cases of disease on a map is a frequently used technique for monitoring the spread of infectious diseases. The dot map drawn by John Snow in the 1850s is possibly the most renowned example,[1] but countless maps exist in offices of the Directorates of Public Health which are charged with monitoring the spread of infectious diseases such as dysentery, meningitis and flu. Dot maps facilitate the search for links between cases. In the case of Snow, dot maps indicated the Broad Street pump as a potential source for the outbreak of cholera. Dot maps of cases of dysentery can elucidate whether the cases are related by residential proximity, by attendance at a particular school, or by some other type of community activity. But dot maps are not restricted to the monitoring of disease. They may be used effectively for monitoring, for example, the uptake of vaccinations or health service usage, or for locating black-spot areas for road traffic accidents. Figure 7.1 shows the sites of road traffic accidents to child pedestrians for one year within a small area of Dundee City. The association between accident location and proximity to schools is clearly demonstrated around several schools shown on the map.

Dot maps of non-infectious diseases, while valuable, are generally not as helpful as dot maps of infectious diseases for establishing the precise cause of disease. Many non-infectious diseases, such as cancer, cardiovascular and cerebrovascular diseases, have multifactorial causes, which makes it

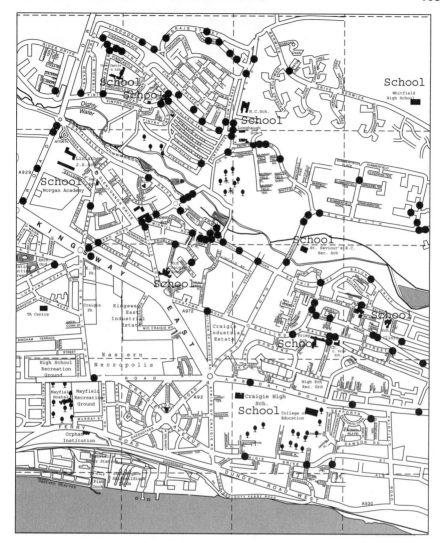

Figure 7.1. Dot map showing locations of fatal road traffic accidents to child pedestrians in Dundee City. Map copyright Geographia Ltd, adapted by permission

extremely difficult to establish cause and effect. When used with such diseases, dot maps are valuable for generating hypotheses about disease causation or for identifying clusters of disease but they do not provide information about specific disease aetiology.

Where the aim is to elucidate causation, the non-infectious diseases which are suited to dot mapping are those which are primarily caused (or triggered) by one factor. For instance a study in Barcelona looked at the onset of an epidemic of asthma by time and by geographical clustering and was able to identify the unloading of soybean in the city's harbour as the cause of the asthma epidemic days.[2] In another study, plotting the residential addresses of cases of lung cancer was one technique by which an association was demonstrated between residential proximity to a steel foundry and lung cancer.[3] (Lung cancer is one of the very few cancers which is caused primarily by a single factor, namely tobacco smoking. It is estimated that tobacco smoking causes 80–85% of lung cancer cases.)

Dot maps require careful interpretation. Because they represent cases spatially, it is essential that the person interpreting the significance of the spatial pattern is familiar with the underlying population structure as this allows an estimate of the population at risk. The interpreter requires local knowledge about the population density, the age and sex structure that the map represents. The higher the population density the higher the number of expected cases. There are several ways in which the demographic characteristics of the population may be assessed. The approach depends on the level of interpretation required. The cases could be converted to incidence rates. But this approach negates the use of a dot map as it forces the use of some (arbitrary) denominator, which is commonly based on a postcode or enumeration district. Another approach is to re-draw the map subdivided into areas that are proportional in size to the population density, the so-called population-based map. Each case, represented by one dot, is placed evenly throughout the area (Figures 7.2a and 7.2b).

It is generally more helpful to monitor the course of diseases with multifactorial causation adjusted for the main confounding factors. Dot maps are not ideal for this purpose as they cannot be adjusted easily. The most typical characteristics, which need to be adjusted for, irrespective of the disease, are the age and sex distributions of a community. Additional factors (such as deprivation indices, smoking and nutritional status) which are disease specific may then need to be considered. A more appropriate way to monitor diseases with multifactorial origins would be to display them using some summary statistic such as the standardized mortality ratio. The standardized mortality ratio is typically adjusted for age and sex but can be adjusted also for disease-specific factors. Where indicated the standardized mortality ratio may be truncated to represent particular groups within a community (for instance, the school ages, working population, young adults, retired population or the very elderly). Of course, caveats concerning the use of SMRs (of [4,6]) must also be considered here.

After deciding whether to use dot maps or adjusted summary statistics for

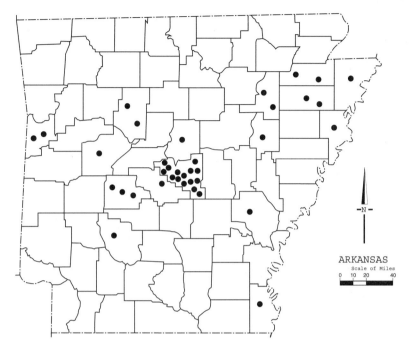

Figure 7.2a. Dot map showing Salmonella cases on a routine geographical map. Redrawn from Dean (1976)[4] by permission

displaying the geographical characteristics of a disease, the next step is to decide on the geographical unit of measurement. To enable a comprehensive review of a health status of a community the data need to be presented in sufficiently small geographical units to allow any potential variations in health to be observed. But the units need to be large enough to enable some sort of statistical interpretation. Health Boards in the UK have access to routinely collected data from the decennial censuses. This information allows the adjustment by many characteristics (for example deprivation indices, ethnicity, age and sex) and is presented at the level of the postcode sector. Table 7.1 describes the hierarchy of units in UK postcodes.

The subdivisions of postcodes are designed to maintain roughly equal populations within each category. For instance postcode units typically represent about 16 households irrespective of which part of the country is represented by the postcode. Because of this principle, postcodes cover very different geographical areas. Densely populated communities will have more postcodes than sparsely populated communities. Postcode sectors

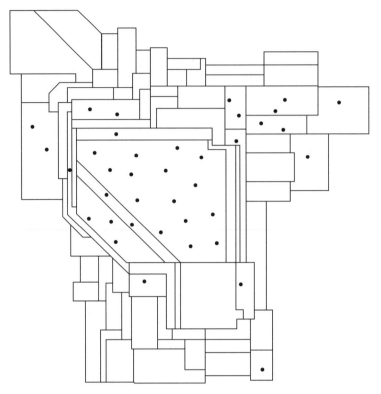

Figure 7.2b. Dot map showing Salmonella cases plotted on a population map. Redrawn from Dean (1976)[4] by permission

Table 7.1   Postcode hierarchy

	Example	Approximate number
Postcode area	FK	1 (i.e there is 1 area starting FK)
Postcode district	FK1	21
Postcode sector	FK1 2	42
Postcode unit	FK1 2ES	> 6000

(Table 7.1) are thus only a reasonable unit for monitoring the health status of communities. By their nature they are more suited to monitoring the health of cities than rural communities. Particular care must be taken if the aim of health monitoring is to assess the impact of pollution on the health of a community. The use of postcode data in such instances may seriously weaken the observed effect because of dilution of the health effect.

ROUTINE MONITORING: ADVANTAGES AND DISADVANTAGES

The routine surveillance of the health of communities has long been considered a desirable development for public health.[5] It is argued that such surveillance would bring several advantages. Firstly, the construction and maintenance of health profiles for each community allows accurate information to be given to a community about its current health status. If an unusual level of morbidity or mortality from a disease were suspected, one of the first questions that would require to be answered would be the health status during the preceding years; routine health surveillance would allow the past health status to be quickly assessed. Secondly, if these health profiles were found to show signs of deterioration, the early warning of any abnormality in mortality (or morbidity) would allow the appropriate measures of public health medicine to be taken, with preventive measures being instituted, assessed and validated with minimal delay. Thirdly, the generation of hypotheses would be facilitated by the knowledge derived from the surveillance of the entire course of an individual epidemic, and also from the more long-term analysis of the geographical distributions of diseases. Finally, detailed knowledge of the health of local communities would allow Health Authorities to provide the quality and quantity of resources appropriate to the local needs.

To be successful, the epidemiological surveillance of communities requires two distinct procedures: the routine surveillance of the whole community; but also the in-depth surveillance of health parameters within the community. The two procedures are complementary, with each contributing information independently. The routine surveillance of the whole community is essential for hypothesis generation and for ascertainment of past and present health status of a community. The in-depth surveillance of health parameters within the community is necessary when trying to identify the causal mechanisms responsible for the unusual levels of mortality or morbidity.

Several techniques can be used to minimize the problem of small numbers. Numbers may be increased by the grouping of several years, or less detailed classifications of diseases may be used. When investigating the health within communities additional sources of data need to be obtained to establish a usable health profile. The additional data collected are dependent on both the suspected cause of the ill health, and the availability of the information. Ultimately, mortality, which is significantly high by chance, can only be distinguished from that which is high from pathogenic causes when pathogenic agents can be found in the environment. This requirement for combined epidemiological and environmental investigations in turn brings the further requirement for environmental techniques to be developed which can be used in conjunction with small-area epidemiology.

Mapping has at least three major roles for the public health medicine specialist. It can be used to map differences in rates of disease; it can be used for mapping and interpreting ecological analyses; and it can be used to map clusters of disease cases, for example, around putative sources of pollution.

MAPPING DIFFERENCES IN RATES

There are numerous examples of mapping in which the main purpose was to compare rates of disease between communities; some of these were reviewed in Chapter 1 and all the atlases which have been published obviously fall into this category.[6–11] Figure 7.3 shows the distribution of standardized mortality ratios for bronchitis, emphysema and asthma in Scotland between 1979 and 1983. It shows quite clearly that the highest mortality was found in the industrialized central belt of Scotland. The strength of this finding was somewhat surprising as it represented deaths 10 years after the passage of the second of the UK's Clean Air Acts.

At a local level, mapping disease within a community health district may also be a helpful way to highlight areas where disease rates are unexpectedly high or low, or where they change over time. Figure 7.4 shows the standardized morbidity ratios for diseases of the nervous system and sense organs for a district in central Scotland during two time periods. The vertical and diagonal areas in Figure 7.4 represent morbidity ratios, which are respectively significantly higher and lower than the standard population. The white areas were neither significantly high nor low. Over the five-year period studied only one district sustained its low morbidity status; two districts improved their poor morbidity and four districts worsened.

Figure 7.5a shows the SMRs for various diseases and Figure 7.5b shows the distribution of various socioeconomic factors for the City of Glasgow. The variability of health within a city is well demonstrated in this example. The inclusion of socioeconomic factors facilitates interpretation of the disease maps. The associations between colorectal and gastric cancer with high unemployment and lower social class contrast with the relation between higher social class and breast cancer. Clearly a statistical assessment of these relations would quantify the nature of the relationship.

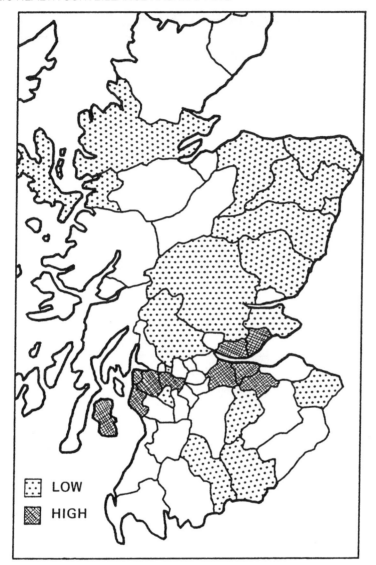

Figure 7.3. SMRs for bronchitis, emphysema and asthma in Scotland between 1979 and 1983. Redrawn from Williams et al. (1987)[20]

Dot maps may also be used to portray the spatial distribution of single events, and this was discussed earlier in this chapter.

Figure 7.6 shows the location of UK fishing vessel losses in Scottish waters between 1973 and 1982. The crosses represent vessels that have foundered and the dot represents other types of loss. Mapping of such costly

99% CONFIDENCE LIMITS

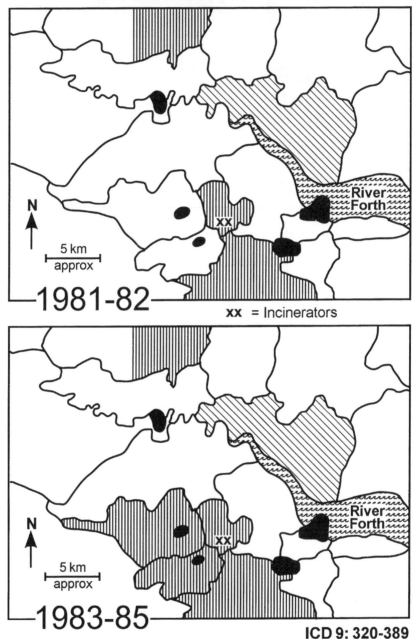

Figure 7.4. Districts in central Scotland with significantly high or low SMRs for CNS diseases

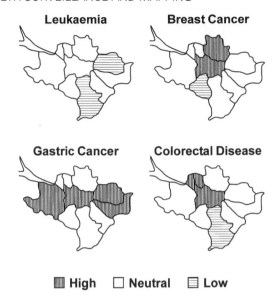

Figure 7.5a. Distribution of SMRs in City of Glasgow

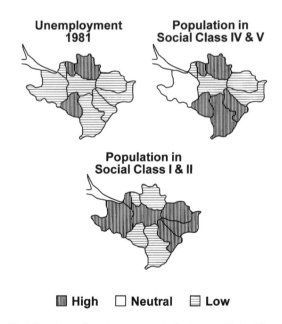

Figure 7.5b. Distribution of socioeconomic factors within City of Glasgow

UK FISHING VESSEL LOSSES IN SCOTTISH WATERS: 1973 - 1982

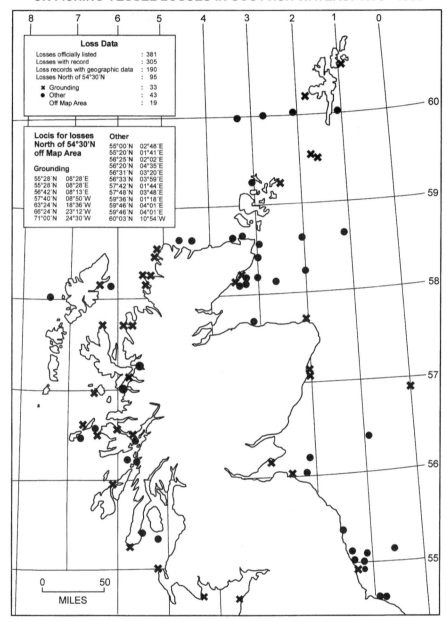

Figure 7.6. UK fishing vessel losses in Scottish waters between 1973 and 1982. Redrawn from Reilly (1987)[6] by permission

events can help by identifying the best locations for search and rescue services.

MAPPING AND INTERPRETING ECOLOGICAL ANALYSES

Mapping may also incorporate aetiological analyses which accommodate explanatory variables. Such studies are sometimes called ecological studies. They are often carried out at an aggregated spatial level. An example of such a study, which is described below, has appeared in a sequence of papers by Bernardinelli and co-workers (see, e.g.[10]).

MALARIA AND INSULIN DEPENDENT DIABETES MELLITUS: AN ECOLOGICAL STUDY

There is scientific merit in studying the association between insulin dependent diabetes mellitus and malaria, since they are both associated with the human leukocyte antigen system. The human leukocyte antigen system is involved in controlling immunological responses, and the association between this system and insulin dependent diabetes mellitus has long been established.[12]

Malaria is the most important natural selective factor on human populations that has been discovered to date.[13] In areas of high endemicity, malaria operates the genetic selection responsible for the influence on the susceptibility to autoimmune diseases.[14] In Sardinia, malaria is known to have selected for some serious hereditary diseases such as β-thalassaemia, Cooley's disease and favism; the latter is caused by a deficiency of glucose-6-phospate dehydrogenase enzyme.[10] Sardinia is therefore particularly suitable for investigating the association between insulin dependent diabetes mellitus and malaria. The incidence of insulin dependent diabetes mellitus in Sardinia is quite atypical of other Mediterranean countries. Sardinia has the second highest incidence in Europe at 33.2 per 100 000 person years; Finland has the highest incidence at 40 per 100 000 person years. A study of 18-year-old military conscripts born between 1936 and 1971 showed that the risk for insulin dependent diabetes mellitus began increasing with the male birth cohort of 1950 and that the increasing trend was much higher than observed in the remainder of Europe.[15] Population genetic studies suggest that, in the plains of Sardinia where malaria had been endemic, some genetic traits were selected to provide greater resistance to the haemolysing action of the Plasmodium vector. In the hilly and mountainous areas, where malaria is almost absent, this adaptation did not occur.[16]

In another study[17] the incidence of insulin dependent diabetes mellitus was obtained from a case registry which had operated in Sardinia since 1989. The incidence data referred to the period 1989–92 and covered the population aged between birth and 29 years. The number of insulin dependent diabetes mellitus cases was available for the 366 communes of Sardinia. Also considered was the number of malaria cases in the communes for the period 1938–40, and the 1936 census populations were available for each commune. The prevalence of malaria between 1938 and 1940 was considered as a covariate, in the model for the calculation of the incidence of insulin dependent diabetes mellitus.

In their modelling approach, the researchers[17] assumed a Poisson likelihood regression model for the counts of insulin dependent diabetes mellitus. But they also found extra-Poisson variation and included a random effect term to allow for this variation. This leads to wider standard errors in the parameter estimates of the regression fit. In addition they found that the malaria prevalence may also include extra noise or error and they modelled also for that effect. They note that: 'in practice, ecological covariates can rarely be observed directly'. Available data may be either imperfect measurements of, or proxies for the true covariate. Sometimes epidemiological data concerning another disease may be used as a proxy variable. For example, to study the geographical variation of heart disease mortality, an important covariate would be the proportion of smokers living in each area. Such specific data on smoking would generally not be available, so the prevalence of lung cancer recorded by the cancer registry for each area might be a useful proxy. The simplest approach to this problem would be to estimate the true covariate from the proxy for each area independently, using the proxy estimate in the ecological regression. When the proxy variable is an accurate measure of the true covariate, this approach would be reasonable. However, when the correspondence between the two is not close, this approach has several disadvantages as not accounting for measurement error causes the point estimate of the regression coefficient to be underestimated and its precision overestimated.

The results of the geographical study of the lagged effect of malaria prevalence and insulin dependent diabetes mellitus suggested a significant negative association between long-term malaria endemicity and diabetes. This suggests that people who live in areas where malaria has been particularly frequent, have a lower risk of insulin dependent diabetes mellitus than those who lived in a low prevalence area in 1938. For instance, the risk of diabetes is considerably lower in the low-lying regions than in the hills and mountains of Sardinia. Malaria endemicity in the low-lying areas could have prevented the onset of insulin dependent diabetes mellitus via stronger selection processes. The 95% credible interval (confidence interval) for the correlation between malaria and insulin dependent diabetes mellitus is -0.812 to -0.182 with a point estimate of nearly -0.6. This interval is wide, but there is some support for a negative relationship.

MAPPING CLUSTERS OF DISEASE CASES

CLUSTER STUDIES

In many applications within public health there is a need to consider whether maps of disease cluster and, if so, where the clusters are located. Often these questions are related to the need for public health authorities to monitor 'unusual' aggregations of disease in localized areas within their area of authority. These concerns may be routine in that there may be a need to provide surveillance of particular diseases and to be aware of any atypical geographical distributions. Intervention or resource reallocation may be the outcome of such surveillance. Another use of such detection is the establishment of aetiological links between some geo-referenced variable and the disease of interest. This linkage may be previously known, or may be as yet undiscovered.

In the analysis of clustering, it is important to distinguish between detection of a clustering tendency over the whole study region (global clustering) and the detection of the locations of clusters (specific clustering). In addition, there is a distinction between the analysis of disease around locations which are known (such as putative sources of hazard, for example incinerators, industrial and domestic chimney flues), and the analysis where the locations of clusters are unknown but need to be estimated. The former is called focused clustering while the latter is termed non-focused clustering.

The analysis of disease incidence around putative health hazards is now an important task assumed by local health authorities. In some cases, a putative hazard is thought by the local community to be a potential health risk, and an alarm is raised, which must be responded to by the health authority. In other cases, a local area is noted to have an elevated disease incidence and so an investigation is initiated into potential contributory factors.

An alternative need in public health and epidemiology is for larger-scale studies of the geographical distribution of clusters and the examination of links between their location and explanatory variables. The outcome of such a study may be the confirmation of aetiological links between, for example, environmental variables and disease risk.

The following briefly describes two examples of such cluster studies: a putative source of hazard example and a large-scale clustering study.

PUTATIVE HEALTH HAZARD EXAMPLE

Following a cluster alarm raised by a local community in Lancashire, UK, an investigation was initiated into the distribution of cancer of the larynx in the vicinity of a waste product incineration facility.

Concern had been expressed that this incinerator could have had an adverse effect upon the respiratory health status of the local area. For the period 1974–83, the larynx cancer case address locations were obtained (Figure 7.7). To allow for the local variation in the population 'at risk' from cancer of the larynx, a realization of all the respiratory cancer cases in the area in the same period was obtained (Figure 7.8). Diggle described the original analysis of this data.[18]

The basis of this approach is examination of the difference between the control and the case local density to find any areas of excess risk. This can

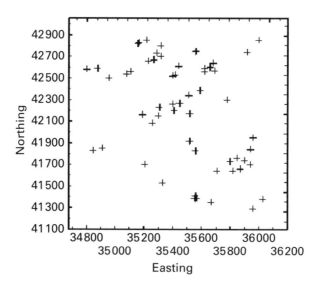

Figure 7.7. Larynx cancer case addresses

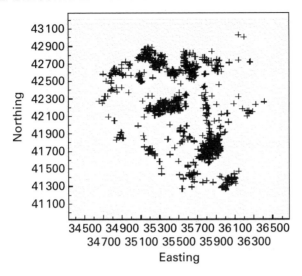

Figure 7.8. Lung cancer (control) cases

be done by simple nonparametric smoothing methods or by applying a model for the relation between the source and the disease of interest. For example, it might be useful to assess if there is a distance–risk relationship. A strong distance decline away from the source might suggest a possible association. Diggle[18] found 'reasonably strong' evidence for such an association in this example, although there is some doubt about the appropriateness of the control disease (which is also a respiratory disease), and the standard errors of the model estimates found were very large.

LARGE-SCALE CLUSTER EXAMPLE

The second example comes from a study of the spatial distribution of congenital birth abnormalities within England.[19] Specifically, the researchers had access to a complete data set of cases of anophthalmia born between 1988 and 1994. The total number of cases was 1658.

A sample of live births for the same period in England was examined. This sample was used as a spatial control for the distribution of congenital abnormality. The control distribution largely reflected the population distribution within England, although it was clearly related to the parental population distribution. The focus of attention was the relation between the spatial distribution of congenital abnormalities and the underlying control distribution. Any excess risk of abnormality might express itself as areas of elevated risk compared to the control distribution. These areas may be regarded as clusters of disease, and it may be of interest to assess whether there are any spatial differences in these clusters and, if so, examine the relation between their distribution and explanatory aetiological variables. Dolk and coworkers[19] examined this example for clustering using a variety of clustering tests.

In that study there was little evidence of localized clustering of abnormalities over the whole study region. However, when particular local study areas were selected, some tests showed significant excess of risk. However, a rural–urban gradient of prevalence was noted, with an increased risk in rural areas. A possible aetiological factor contributing to this effect was pesticide exposure, but there was little evidence to support this link. An alternative environmental factor considered was maternal infection during pregnancy. There was no evidence found for a link between socioeconomic deprivation and abnormalities.

The growing availability and affordability of desktop computers has greatly changed the work potential of the typical public health specialist. The ubiquity of computers has resulted in the increased accessibility of data sets, such as census data, routine health statistics and ad hoc databases. This has been paralleled by an enormous increase in the availability and sophistication of user friendly software that has been specifically designed to allow the visual representation of data. Moreover, more recently, the software has been developed to incorporate basic analytical tools. Disparate data sets can be easily assimilated on to one map, and associations that would otherwise remain obscured in complex tables or text can become immediately apparent. The Appendix describes some of the software currently available.

REFERENCES

1. Snow J (1936). Snow on cholera: being a reprint of two papers. London: The Commonwealth Fund.
2. Antó JM, Sunyer J, Rodriguez-Roisin R, Suarez-Cervera M and Vazquez L (1989). Community outbreaks of asthma associated with inhalation of soybean dust. *New England Journal of Medicine* **320**: 1097–102.
3. Lloyd OL (1978). Respiratory cancer clustering associated with localised industrial air pollution. *Lancet* **i**: 318–20.

SUMMARY

1. Disease mapping plays an important role in the monitoring of a community's health.
2. Epidemiological surveillance should be a two-step procedure. First, routine surveillance of the whole community. Secondly, indepth surveillance of selected health parameters.
3. Mapping has at least four major roles for public health specialists:
   (i) Monitoring the spread of infectious diseases in order to identify the cause of the infection.
   (ii) Monitoring health service usage such as the uptake of vaccination or the use of community care services.
   (iii) Mapping of the non-infectious diseases is valuable for generating hypotheses about disease causation or for identifying clusters of disease.
   (iv) Mapping exercises can incorporate ecological analyses which can adjust for explanatory variables.

4. Dean AG (1976). Population-based spot maps: an epidemiologic technique. *American Journal of Public Health* **66**(10): 988–9.
5. England PH (1988). *The Report of the Committee of Inquiry into the Future Development of the Public Health Function.* London: HMSO.
6. Lloyd OL, Williams FLR, Berry WG and Florey CduV (eds) (1987). *An Atlas of Mortality in Scotland.* London: Croom Helm.
7. Kemp I, Boyle P, Smans M and Muir C (eds) (1985). *Atlas of Cancer in Scotland 1975–80: Incidence and Epidemiological Perspective.* Lyon: IARC Scientific Publications.
8. Gardner MJ, Winter PD and Barker DJP (1984). *Atlas of Disease Mortality from Selected Diseases in England and Wales 1968–1978.* Chichester: Wiley.
9. Howe GM (1963). *National Atlas of Disease Mortality in the United Kingdom.* London: Nelson.
10. Bernardinelli L, Maida A, Marinoni A and Clayton D (1994). *Atlas of Cancer Mortality in Sardinia, 1983–87.* FATMA-CNR.
11. Leukaemia Research Fund (1990). *Leukaemia and Lymphoma: an Atlas of Distribution within Areas of England and Wales 1984–1988.* Leukaemia Research Fund.
12. Todd J, Bell J and McDevitt H (1990). A molecular basis for genetic susceptibility in insulin dependent diabetes mellitus. *Trends in Genetics* **4**: 129–34.

13. Jacob CO (1992). Tumor necrosis factor α in autoimmunity: pretty girl or cold witch? *Immunology Today* **13**: 122–5.
14. Wilson AG and Duff GW (1995). Genetic traits in common diseases supports the adage that autoimmunity is the price paid for erradicating infectious disease. *British Medical Journal* **310**: 1482–3.
15. Muntoni S and Songini M (1992). High incidence rates of IDDM in Sardinia. *Diabetes Care* **15**: 1317–22.
16. Piazza A, Mayr W and Contu L (1985), Amoroso Aea. Genetic population of four Sardinian villages. *Annals of Human Genetics* **4**: 47–63.
17. Bernardinelli L, Pascutto C, Best NG and Gilks W (1997). Disease mapping with errors in covariates. *Statistics in Medicine* **16**: 741–52.
18. Diggle P (1990). Modelling the prevalence of cancer of the larnyx in part of Lancashire: a new methodology for spatial epidemiology. In: Thomas RW (ed.). *Spatial Epidemiology*: London: Pion, pp. 35–47.
19. Dolk H, Bushby A, Armstrong B and Walls PH (1998). Geographical variation in anopthalmia and micropthalmia in England, 1988–1994. *British Medical Journal* **317**: 905–10.
20. Williams FLR, Lloyd OL and Berry WG (1987). Mortality from nonmalignant respiratory disease in Scotland between 1959 and 1983. *Ambio* **16**: 206–10.

Appendix: Software for Disease Mapping

A wide variety of software is now available to provide assessment of spatial data. This ranges from modules for spatial statistical analysis in, for example, S-Plus, to complete Geographical Information Systems (GIS) such as MAPINFO or ARCVIEW which usually do not have spatial statistical capabilities. The software available can be conveniently divided into two basic types: firstly, spatial statistical tools, which usually are not integrated into a general GIS environment, and, secondly, general packages which allow users to manipulate and display geo-referenced data.

SPATIAL STATISTICAL TOOLS

A number of packages and modules within packages now provide access to spatial statistical procedures. The most notable of these are the Spatial module of S-Plus, and the SPLANCS system (University of Lancaster), which also interfaces with S-Plus. S-Plus is a widely available statistical package which is currently provided only on Unix and Windows formats, but not in other mainframe operating systems. Hence, the availability of these modules is limited by hardware configuration. The Spatial module provides basic descriptive spatial analysis measures, Kriging estimators and point process related methods. It does not provide a general modelling capability in applications in spatial epidemiology. The SPLANCS package, which is a set of S-Plus functions, does provide some specialist tools for the analysis of point event data in both space and space–time (e.g. kernel smoothing), and functions for analysis of putative hazard problems and other clustering problems, based on methods developed by workers at

Lancaster University. The S-Plus package has a file transfer link with the GIS ARCVIEW also. However, none of these systems provide an integrated spatial data analysis platform, which can be used easily to carry out data manipulation and analysis.

Some packages have been developed specifically for the analysis of small-area count data and these sometimes have improved data display and management facilities. DISMAPWIN[1] is a general purpose package which can display small-area count maps and provides a range of further analysis steps, including computation of SMRs, empirical Bayes estimation of relative risks, mixture analysis and covariate adjustment. BEAM has also been developed to provide a platform for Bayesian ecological analysis of mapped data, and does provide display and manipulation functions as well as statistical mapping procedures. It is also possible to use the general BUGS MCMC software[2] to analyse hierarchical models for mapped data, but GIS facilities are not currently available. The MLn software developed by the multi-level modelling project,[3] can also be used to analyse hierarchical models, although based on normal approximations to distributions in the hierarchy.

For certain tasks, such as evaluating test statistics, some software is available, and software to provide a range of testing possibilities is currently being developed. For example, in cluster testing, SatScan software for testing spatial and spatio-temporal clustering via scan statistics, is available for Windows 95/NT.[4] Stat! is a general package providing analysis of clustering of health events,[5] which has Windows 95/NT versions in development. Other software from the same source are Gamma, GBAS and GeoMed which are funded by the National Cancer Institute (USA), and deal with specific aspects of spatial analysis. GeoMed in particular, deals with general and focused clustering tests and is currently in development. The CDC (Centre for Disease Control, Atlanta, USA) has also developed a programme entitled Cluster which can carry out a range of cluster tests. The development of cluster testing software within the GIS package MAPINFO is also underway at CDC.

In addition to purpose-designed software for specific tasks, a number of general purpose statistical packages can be employed in some applications. For likelihood models of the Poisson process or Poisson-count type, packages such as GLIM, SPLUS or BMDP could be used in applications to putative health hazards or in general ecological modelling.[6,7] However, when random effect models are employed, particularly those including correlated heterogeneity, often recourse must be made to Bayesian or multi-level software. The packages BEAM and BUGS can provide a general hierarchical modelling framework, but do not provide any flexibility when correlation structures are to be modified, and hence emphasize the Bayesian rather than spatial aspects of the modelling process. Similar comments also apply to the MLn software package. Approximations other than those used in the MLn software can also be accommodated, if in simple forms, by GLIM.

GEOGRAPHICAL INFORMATION SYSTEMS

There are now a large variety of commercially available software packages which provide display and manipulation facilitites for geo-referenced data. These packages are usually referred to as Geographical Information Systems (GIS). The fundamental ingredient of these packages is the idea of map layers which contain different information about the mapped area. For example, in one layer might be held the tract boundaries of census small areas, while in another layer some additional information relating to each tract can be stored and displayed: for example, census small-area labels or SMRs or crude counts. Each layer can be manipulated interactively (edited) to provide a composite map. In addition, some packages also provide facilities for selection of sub-areas or arbitrary transect displays. The types of display available on the commonest packages are often limited to types of thematic map (choropleth, dot maps, etc.), and often contour or interpolation facilities are crude or not available in the basic package. In addition, the ability to handle (point) objects, in a reasonably sophisticated manner, has only recently become available. One major drawback of current systems is their lack of spatial statistical tools for analysis of spatial data. It is widely regarded that the commonest GIS packages in use currently are MapInfo[TM] and ArcView[TM], and we focus here on these packages. These packages have been developing over the last 15–20 years and have different market orientations. MapInfo has as its focus the manipulation of polygons and their associated data. Hence, small-area tract information is well suited to this format, and many business-related applications can be developed with this package. It is also possible to use MapInfo for the analysis of (point) object data via add-on software (e.g. Vertical Mapper[TM]), which can provide interpolated surfaces and compute tesselations. On the other hand, ArcView has focused on continuous surface modelling and mapping functionality, and therefore finds considerable use in land use assessment and a wide range of environmental applications. Both packages have links to statistical software packages and to each other via data transfer facilities, and there are additional facilities which allow user programming of GIS itself. However, these packages still await the incorporation of spatial statistical tools.

SOFTWARE AVAILABILITY AND WEB SITES

DISMAPWIN

http://ftp.ukbf.fu-berlin.de/sozmed/DismapWin.html
A downloadable version of DISMAPWIN is available from this web site. It includes a variety of example maps and a limited help facility.

SPLANCS

http://www.maths.lancs.ac.uk/~rowlings/Splancs
This package is available in two versions and can be obtained from the Department of Mathematics, University of Lancaster, Baillrigg, Lancaster, UK. There is a small charge for the software.

BUGS and BEAM

http://www.mrc-bsu.cam.ac.uk
The package BUGS (Bayesian Inference using Gibbs Sampling) is available in a windows version as shareware (WINBUGS) from the MRC Unit of Biostatistics, Cambridge University, which maintains this site. BEAM is also available from this location.

MLnWIN

http://www.ioe.ac.uk/multilevel
A windows version of the MLn software package is available as MLnWIN. This can be purchased from the Multi-Level Modelling Project, Institute of Education, University of London, London, UK.

SATSCAN

Email to martink@cortex.uchc.edu
This is available as shareware from Professor Martin Kulldorff, Department of Statistics, School of Public Health, University of Connecticut, USA.

Stat! , Gamma, GBAS, SPACESTAT, GST and GeoMed

These packages are available from Biomedware Inc., 516 North State Street, Ann Arbor, Michigan, 48104-1236, USA, for a small charge.
http://www.biomedware.com

MapInfo

This commercial GIS package is available from a variety of software

stockists and further information about local dealers can be obtained from MAPINFO at http://www.mapinfo.com
or email to
sales@mapinfo.com

ArcView

This GIS package is obtainable from ESRI, 380 New York Street, Redlands, California, 92373-8100, USA
web site: http://www.esri.com/software/arcview
or http://www.esriuk.com/

REFERENCES

1. Schlattman P and Bohning D (1993). Mixture models and disease mapping. *Statistics in Medicine.* **12**: 1943–50.
2. Pascutto C, Bernardinelli L, Best NG and Gilks WR (1996). Ecological regression with errors in covariates: an application. Statistical Modelling: *Proceedings of the 11th International Workshop on Statistical Modelling.* Forcina A, Marchetti GM, Hatzinger R and Galmacci G (eds). Graphos, Citta di Castello, pp. 299–307.
3. Langford I, Leyland A, Rashbash J, Goldstein H, McDonald A-L and Bentham G (1999). Modelling of area-based health data. In: Lawson AB, Biggeri A, Boehning D, Lesaffre E, Viel JF and Bertollini R (eds). *Disease Mapping and Risk Assessment for Public Health Decision Making.* Wiley, pp. 17–227.
4. Kulldorff M and Nagarwalla N (1995). Spatial disease clusters: detection and inference. *Statistics in Medicine.* **14**: 799–810.
5. Jacquez G (1994). *Stat!: Statistical Software for the Clustering of Health Events.* Ann Arbor: Biomedware.
6. Lawson AB (1993). On the analysis of mortality events around a prespecified fixed point. *Journal of the Royal Statistical Society A* **156**: 363–77.
7. Lawson AB and Williams FLR (1994). Armadale: a case study in environmental epidemiology. *Journal of the Royal Statistical Society A* **157**: 285–298.

Glossary

A posteriori inference   Inference made where the subject of inference has been raised outwith properly structured scientific investigation. Bias may arise due to this selection.

Atomistic fallacy   The bias introduced when the results of statistical inference, based on individual level studies, is applied to aggregated data units.

Bonferonni's inequality   Control of the overall error rate in multiple comparisons, by adjustment of individual comparison error rates.

Cohort study   A study design which investigates disease *prospectively*. Study subjects are identified and followed up over a period of time in order to monitor the occurrence and nature of disease. The prospective design allows information on confounding variables to be accurately recorded.

Correlated heterogeneity   Unobserved variables can induce extra variation (heterogeneity) in disease rates and this variation can appear to be spatially correlated.

Denominator data   Data that are used on the bottom of an equation such as

$$\frac{\text{Number of deaths from heart disease in Town A }[\textit{numerator data}]}{\text{Population in town A }[\textit{denominator data}]}$$

Dot map   A map of cases of disease where the locations (usually residential) are represented as dot symbols.

Ecological fallacy   The bias introduced when the results of statistical inference, based on aggregate data, are applied at the individual level.

Edge effect   The proximity to the boundary of a study region can induce bias in statistical inference for the study region.

Enumeration district   A census district in the UK, within which an enumerator collects census data within one day.

Focused clustering   The analysis of the clustering tendency of disease around a fixed (known) location.

Incidence   The number of *new* cases of disease which occur in a specified time period and in a specified population.

Non-focused clustering   The analysis of the clustering tendency of disease around unspecified (unknown) cluster locations.

Numerator data   Data that are used on the top of an equation such as

$$\frac{\text{Number of deaths from heart disease in Town A } [\textit{numerator data}]}{\text{Population in town A } [\textit{denominator data}]}$$

Prevalence   The number of *new and exisiting* cases of disease which occur in a specified time period and in a specified population.

Random effects   Unobserved factors/variates can lead to extra variation in disease maps. These effects can be included in the analysis of the map using random effects, which add extra-variation to the analysis.

Relative risk   The ratio of the incidence of disease in the *exposed* population to the incidence in the *non-exposed* population.

Standardized Mortality Ratio (SMR)   The ratio of the observed mortality in a community to the expected mortality in that community according to experience of some standard population.

Uncorrelated heterogeneity   As for Correlated heterogeneity except the unobserved variation is spatially uncorrelated.

Index

Index compiled by Anne McCarthy